Enola K. Proctor
Nancy Morrow-Howell
Arlene Stiffman
Editors

Mental Health Services and Sectors of Care

Mental Health Services and Sectors of Care has been co-published simultaneously as *Journal of Social Service Research*, Volume 25, Number 3 1999.

Pre-publication
REVIEWS,
COMMENTARIES,
EVALUATIONS . . .

"**I**n an era characterized by a lack of information about services provided, especially to youth with severe emotional disorders and confusion stemming from the growth of managed care, THIS . . . IS TIMELY. It provides new information from six methodologically rigorous studies based in sites spanning a wide geographical range . . ."

Barbara J. Burns, PhD
Professor and Director
Service Effectiveness Research Program
Department of Psychiatry
and Behavioral Sciences
Duke University Medical Center
Durham, North Carolina

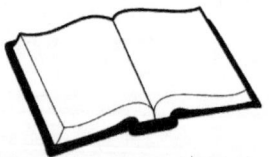

Mental Health Services and Sectors of Care

Mental Health Services and Sectors of Care has been co-published simultaneously as *Journal of Social Service Research*, Volume 25, Number 3 1999.

The *Journal of Social Service Research* Monographic "Separates"

Below is a list of "separates," which in serials librarianship means a special issue simultaneously published as a special journal issue or double-issue *and* as a "separate" hardbound monograph. (This is a format which we also call a "DocuSerial.")

"Separates" are published because specialized libraries or professionals may wish to purchase a specific thematic issue by itself in a format which can be separately cataloged and shelved, as opposed to purchasing the journal on an on-going basis. Faculty members may also more easily consider a "separate" for classroom adoption.

"Separates" are carefully classified separately with the major book jobbers so that the journal tie-in can be noted on new book order slips to avoid duplicate purchasing.

You may wish to visit Haworth's website at . . .

http://www.haworthpressinc.com

. . . to search our online catalog for complete tables of contents of these separates and related publications.

You may also call 1-800-HAWORTH (outside US/Canada: 607-722-5857), or Fax: 1-800-895-0582 (outside US/Canada: 607-771-0012), or e-mail at:

getinfo@haworthpressinc.com

Mental Health Services and Sectors of Care, edited by Enola K. Proctor, MSSW, PhD, Nancy Morrow-Howell, MSW, PhD, and Arlene Stiffman, PhD (Vol. 25, No. 3, 1999). *" . . . Contributes data that will help move forward the research base in a field which has traditionally lacked evidence-based understanding."* (Barbara J. Burns, PhD, Professor and Director, Service Effectiveness Research Program, Department of Psychiatry and Behavioral Sciences, Duke University Medical Center, Durham, North Carolina)

Social Work Research with Minority and Oppressed Populations: Methodological Issues and Innovations, edited by Miriam Potocky, PhD, and Antoinette Y. Rodgers-Farmer, PhD (Vol. 23, No. 3/4, 1998). *"This splendid book is a much-needed contribution to the social work literature. . . . It is a major breakthrough, setting a path that compels practitioners and especially social work researchers to follow."* (Bogart Leashore, PhD, Dean and Professor, School of Social Work, Hunter College, New York, New York)

Research on Social Work and Disasters, edited by Calvin L. Streeter, PhD, and Susan A. Murty, PhD (Vol. 22, No. 1/2, 1996). *"A superb job in bringing together this collection of disaster research chapters. This compilation of studies represents the state of the art for social work disaster research."* (Michael J. Zakour, PhD, Assistant Professor and Director, Disaster & Volunteerism Research Center, School of Social Work, Tulane University, New Orleans, Louisiana)

Single-System Designs in the Social Services: Issues and Options for the 1990s, edited by Martin Bloom, PhD (Vol. 18, No. 1/2, 1994). *"A State-of-the-Art book on the expanding applications of this innovative methodology to diverse areas of practice."* (Bruce A. Thyer, PhD, Professor of Social Work, University of Georgia)

Quantitative Methods in Social Work: State of the Art, edited by David F. Gillespie, PhD, and Charles Glisson, PhD (Vol. 16, No. 1/2/3, 1993). *"Reviews the quantitative methods used by researchers in social work, describing the theory, methodology, and issues and techniques of specific applications."* (SciTech Book News)

Advances in Group Work Research, edited by Sheldon D. Rose, PhD, and Aaron M. Brower, PhD (Vol. 13, No. 2, 1990). *"In this comprehensive overview of the state of the art in the field, group workers and social scientists explore group research issues."*

Progress in Behavioral Social Work, edited by Bruce A. Thyer, PhD, and Walter W. Hudson, PhD (Vol. 10, No. 2/3/4, 1988). *"Fills a major gap in the literature on behavioural social work by not restricting itself merely to defining what behavioural social work is and how it has evolved, but by providing illustrations of its applications to different problem-areas ranging from the medical to the psychiatric.'' (The Indian Journal of Social Work)*

Burnout Among Social Workers, edited by David F. Gillespie, PhD (Vol. 10, No. 1, 1987). *"This timely book provides a highly significant contribution to our understanding of burnout. Helping professionals, administrators, and researchers will find this book to be a valuable source of empirical findings on the phenomenon of burnout.'' (Arnold Barnes, PhD, Assistant Professor, School of Social Work, Grambling State University)*

Single-System Research Designs, edited by Martin Bloom, PhD (Vol. 3, No. 1, 1979). *"A concise and readable volume that bridges the gap between social work research and social research in general.''*

New Models of Social Service Research, edited by Edwin J. Thomas (Vol. 2, No. 1, 1979). *"A comprehensive review, synthesis, and analysis of models of applied research in the social and human services.''*

Mental Health Services and Sectors of Care has been co-published simultaneously as *Journal of Social Service Research*™, Volume 25, Number 3 1999.

First published 1999 by
The Haworth Press, Inc.

Published 2014 by Routledge
2 Park Square, Milton Park, Abingdon, Oxfordshire OX14 4RN
711 Third Avenue, New York, NY 10017

Routledge is an imprint of the Taylor & Francis Group, an informa business
First issued in paperback 2014

Cover design by Thomas J. Mayshock Jr.

Library of Congress Cataloging-in-Publication Data

Mental health services and sectors of care / Enola K. Proctor, Nancy Morrow-Howell, Arlene Stiffman.
    p. cm.
    "Has been co-published simultaneously as Journal of social service research, volume 25, Number 3, 1999."
    Includes bibliographical references and index.
    ISBN 978-0-7890-0760-5 (hbk) ISBN 978-1-1380-0240-1 (pbk)
    1. Mental health services Miscellanea. 2. Crisis intervention (Mental health services) Miscellanea. I. Proctor, Enola Knisley. II. Morrow-Howell, Nancy. III. Stiffman, Arlene Rubin, 1941- .
RA790.5.M47 1999
362.2–dc21   99-17012
                                                                CIP

Mental Health Services and Sectors of Care

Enola K. Proctor
Nancy Morrow-Howell
Arlene Stiffman
Editors

Mental Health Services and Sectors of Care has been co-published simultaneously as *Journal of Social Service Research,* Volume 25, Number 3 1999.

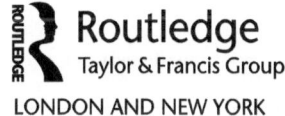

Routledge
Taylor & Francis Group

LONDON AND NEW YORK

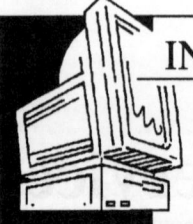

INDEXING & ABSTRACTING

Contributions to this publication are selectively indexed or abstracted in print, electronic, online, or CD-ROM version(s) of the reference tools and information services listed below. This list is current as of the copyright date of this publication. See the end of this section for additional notes.

- *Abstracts in Social Gerontology: Current Literature on Aging*

- *Applied Social Sciences Index & Abstracts (ASSIA) (Online: ASSI via Data-Star) (CDRom: ASSIA Plus)*

- *Behavioral Medicine Abstracts*

- *BUBL Information Service, an Internet-based Information Service for the UK higher education community*

- *caredata CD: the social and community care database*

- *CNPIEC Reference Guide: Chinese National Directory of Foreign Periodicals*

- *Criminal Justice Abstracts*

- *Current Contents . . . . see: Institute for Scientific Information*

- *Family Studies Database (online and CD/ROM)*

- *Human Resources Abstracts (HRA)*

- *IBZ International Bibliography of Periodical Literature*

- *Index to Periodical Articles Related to Law*

- *Institute for Scientific Information*

- *Mental Health Abstracts (online through DIALOG)*

- *National Center for Chronic Disease Prevention & Health Promotion (NCCDPHP)*

(continued)

- *National Clearinghouse on Child Abuse & Neglect*

- *NIAAA Alcohol and Alcohol Problems Science Database (ETOH)*

- *PASCAL, c/o Institute de L'Information Scientifique et Technique*

- *Psychological Abstracts (PsycINFO)*

- *Social Planning/Policy & Development Abstracts (SOPODA)*

- *Social Science Citation Index .... see: Institute for Scientific Information*

- *Social Work Abstracts*

- *Sociological Abstracts (SA)*

Special Bibliographic Notes related to special journal issues (separates) and indexing/abstracting:

- indexing/abstracting services in this list will also cover material in any "separate" that is co-published simultaneously with Haworth's special thematic journal issue or DocuSerial. Indexing/abstracting usually covers material at the article/chapter level.
- monographic co-editions are intended for either non-subscribers or libraries which intend to purchase a second copy for their circulating collections.
- monographic co-editions are reported to all jobbers/wholesalers/approval plans. The source journal is listed as the "series" to assist the prevention of duplicate purchasing in the same manner utilized for books-in-series.
- to facilitate user/access services all indexing/abstracting services are encouraged to utilize the co-indexing entry note indicated at the bottom of the first page of each article/chapter/contribution.
- this is intended to assist a library user of any reference tool (whether print, electronic, online, or CD-ROM) to locate the monographic version if the library has purchased this version but not a subscription to the source journal.
- individual articles/chapters in any Haworth publication are also available through the Haworth Document Delivery Service (HDDS).

Mental Health Services and Sectors of Care

CONTENTS

Introduction   1
Enola K. Proctor

Youth Entering an Emergency Shelter Care Facility: Prior
Involvement in Juvenile Justice and Mental Health Systems   5
Alan J. Litrownik
Heather N. Taussig
John A. Landsverk
Ann F. Garland

Physician-Patient Gender and the Recognition and Treatment
of Depression in Primary Care   21
Lee W. Badger
Michael Berbaum
Patricia A. Carney
Allen J. Dietrich
Mary Owen
John T. Stem

Reactivity and Responsiveness in Children's Service Systems   41
William R. Nugent
Charles Glisson

The Dynamics of Interagency Collaboration: How Linkages
Develop for Child Welfare and Juvenile Justice Sectors
in a System of Care Demonstration   61
Jeanne C. Rivard
Matthew C. Johnsen
Joseph P. Morrissey
Barbara E. Starrett

Youth and Provider Perspectives on Social Service Providers'
Roles in Mental Health Services   83
    Arlene Rubin Stiffman
    Diane Elze
    Eric Hadley-Ives
    Sharon Johnson

Depression Treatment and Cost Offset for Rural Community
Residents with Depression   99
    Mingliang Zhang
    Kathryn M. Rost
    John C. Fortney

Index   111

ABOUT THE EDITORS

Enola K. Proctor, MSSW, PhD, is Frank J. Bruno Professor of Social Work Research in the George Warren Brown School of Social Work at Washington University in St. Louis, MO. Dr. Proctor directs the Center for Mental Health Services Research and a PhD training program in mental health services research, both funded by the National Institute of Mental Health. Her research in health and mental health services has been supported by grants from the Agency for Health Care Policy and Research, the National Institute of Mental Health, the AARP Andrus Foundation, and the American Heart Association. Dr. Proctor's work has appeared in several social work, health, and mental health journals, and she is co-author of *Race, Gender, and Class: Guidelines for Practice with Individuals, Families, and Groups*. In addition, Dr. Proctor received the Washington University Distinguished Faculty Award in 1992, the National Association of Social Workers' Presidential Award for Excellence in Research in 1994, the Mental Health Professional of the Year award from the St. Louis Alliance for the Mentally Ill in 1997 and the George Warren Brown Distinguished Faculty Award in 1998.

Nancy Morrow-Howell, MSW, PhD, is Associate Professor in the George Warren Brown School of Social Work at Washington University in St. Louis, MO, where she teaches gerontology as well as research courses. Her research interests are in community services and mental health services to elders in need. In addition, Dr. Morrow-Howell is an investigator with the Center for Mental Health Services Research at Washington University. She is co-author of "Adequacy of Care: The Concept and Its Measurement" and "Evaluating an Intervention for Elders at Increased Risk of Suicide," both in the journal *Research on Social Work Practice*. Dr. Morrow-Howell received Distinguished Faculty Awards from the George Warren Brown School of Social Work and Washington University in 1997.

Arlene Stiffman, PhD, is Professor in the George Warren Brown School of Social Work at Washington University in St. Louis, MO, where she is Associate Director of the Center for Mental Health Services Research, funded by the (NIMH) National Institute of Mental Health. She has been the Principal Investigator of several funded studies of adolescent mental health/behavioral problems and service use. Her publications have focused on multisector services and on the person-environment relationship, two of which earned her awards, Best Paper of 1995 by *Health Education Quarterly* and Best Paper in the Social Science Category at the Seventh International Conference on AIDS in 1991.

Introduction

Findings from the Epidemiologic Catchment Area (ECA) studies, supported by the National Institute of Mental Health, demonstrate not only the prevalence of mental disorder (Regier & Robins, 1991), but also the tremendous gap between need and service. Few adults, children, and adolescents with mental disorder receive any care. Only about one in five of those who do receive care are treated by mental health specialists (Katendahl & Realini, 1995; Regier et al., 1993; Coyne et al., 1994; Shulbert et al., 1995; Hoagwood, 1994; Regier et al., 1982). ECA researchers concluded that the U.S. mental health service delivery system comprises multiple sectors, including specialty mental health, general medical physicians, human (social) services, and involuntary self-help (Regier et al., 1993). Most care, particularly for such vulnerable groups as older adults, minorities, and children and adolescents, is provided through a complex and uncoordinated "de facto" system of care (Regier et al., 1978, p. 686).

This volume addresses the challenges of mental health service delivery in these multiple systems of care. Although prior research indicates that medical and social services play an important role in the care of those with mental disorder, we know very little about the contribution of various sectors (Regier et al., 1993) in ensuring adequate care. Studies are needed that delve into the "de facto" system of care, conceptual and methodological challenges to such research notwithstanding. The articles assembled here make important contributions on both the substantive and methodological fronts. Each demonstrates that mental disorders are present within and have potential to burden nonspecialty care, particularly the medical and social service sectors.

Two articles highlight the importance of detection and referral by nonspecialty providers. Findings of Stiffman, Elze, Hadley-Ives, and Johnson underscore the pivotal role of social service providers in the identification, treatment, and referral of persons needing mental health care. Although multiple profes-

[Haworth co-indexing entry note]: "Introduction." Proctor, Enola K. Co-published simultaneously in *Journal of Social Service Research* (The Haworth Press, Inc.) Vol. 25, No. 3, 1999, pp. 1-4; and: *Mental Health Services and Sectors of Care* (ed: Enola K. Proctor, Nancy Morrow-Howell, and Arlene Stiffman) The Haworth Press, Inc., 1999, pp. 1-4. Single or multiple copies of this article are available for a fee from The Haworth Document Delivery Service [1-800-342-9678, 9:00 a.m. - 5:00 p.m. (EST). E-mail address: getinfo@haworthpressinc.com].

sionals were involved in serving troubled youth, social service providers served more such youngsters than did all other professionals. Contact with a social service professional was a significant predictor of subsequent mental health care for adolescents. Within primary medical care, the detection of mental disorder among primary care physicians has long been a focus of concern. The findings of Badger, Berbaum, Carney, Dietrich, Owen, and Stem suggest that physicians may be doing a better job detecting and responding to depression than in earlier years. Nonetheless, evidence of significant gender differences, with male physicians failing to discuss and recommend depression treatment as often among male patients, is troubling. These two studies highlight the importance of continued research and professional training around the gate-keeping role of medical and social service providers. Their role is key in reducing the gap between mental health needs and services.

Focusing more broadly at the service system, Nugent and Glisson address the important question, "How responsive are social service sectors to mental health problems?" Their findings indicate that at least the system they studied—the Tennessee child custody system—not only fails to respond to child mental health needs but also actually attempts to avoid such problems through service refusals. Clearly, nonspecialty sectors need to either provide services appropriate to the mental disorder so prevalent among the clients or link clients with needed mental health services. The findings of Litrownik, Taussig, Landsverk, and Garland shed light on the complicated routes to mental health care. They challenge the assumption of a unidirectional path to care by demonstrating that involvement with the mental health specialty sector both precedes and follows involvement with the criminal justice and child welfare system. They further demonstrate that persons with mental disorder receive services from multiple sources of care, sequentially or simultaneously. Rivard, Johnsen, Morrissey, and Starrett report findings of a system-level intervention designed to integrate service delivery across sectors for children with serious emotional disturbances. Following the intervention, agencies evidenced incremental growth in cooperation. Future studies are needed to determine whether such cooperation actually helps link clients to needed care.

Studies by Nugent and Glisson, Litrownik et al., and Zhang, Rost, and Fortney add to evidence that mental disorder burdens social and medical systems of care. These studies show that mental disorder burdens the process of care (e.g., multiple placements, ejection from care for children in custody), is associated with less favorable outcomes (e.g., placement with non-relatives rather than the more desirable family reunification), and raises costs (e.g., greater cost for treating physical problems in lieu of depression treatment expenditures). Most important, Zhang et al. demonstrate that treating mental disorder results in cost-savings in nonspecialty (general medical) care.

These articles make important methodological contributions to mental health services research, as well. The studies utilized prospective (Stiffman et al., Badger et al., Nugent & Glisson) design, methods of analysis appropriate for longitudinal data (Stiffman et al., Rivard et al.), and randomized design (Badger et al.). Zhang et al. measure service use and cost data by obtaining and abstracting records from health providers and third party payers.

Research examining provision of mental health services within general medical sectors has been a major program emphasis of the NIMH (Taube & Burns, 1988). We need a comparable research agenda within the social service sector, and social work researchers are well positioned to lead such an agenda. Social work was designated as one of the four core mental health professions in the federal legislation establishing the NIMH, and social workers are the largest professional group of mental health service providers (Redick et al., 1992). Social workers play a major role in all four sectors: specialty mental health, general medicine, social services, and informal care. Social work has singular familiarity with service delivery systems, referral processes, and the range of community services. Social workers may be the best-informed professionals about the needy and under-served. Yet social work's contribution to research in mental health has long lagged behind its service contribution, with unfortunate consequences for practice-relevant knowledge.

The growing involvement of social work researchers in externally funded mental health research, in NIMH-supported research centers, and on interdisciplinary research teams enhances their ability to make significant contributions to mental health services research. Two studies reported in this collection—Stiffman et al. and Nugent and Glisson—were conducted within NIMH-funded Social Work Research Development Centers, at Washington University and University of Tennessee, respectively. Other studies (Zhang et al., Rivard et al., Litrownik et al.) were supported by other types of NIMH research centers. Social work research on multi-sector delivery of mental health services will become even more pressing as managed care is expected to further restrict access to specialty mental health care.

Enola K. Proctor

REFERENCES

Coyne, J.C., Fechner-Bates, S. & Schwenk, T.L. (1994). Prevalence, nature, and comorbidity of depressive disorders in primary care. *General Hospital Psychiatry, 16*, 267-276.

Hoagwood, K. (1994). Introduction to the special section: Issues in designing and implementing studies in non-mental health care sectors. *Journal of Clinical Child Psychology, 23*(2), 114-120.

Katendahl, D.A., & Realini, J.P. (1995). Where do panic attack sufferers seek care? *Journal of Family Practice, 40*(3), 237-243.

Redick, R.W., Witkin, M.J., Atay, J.E. & Manderscheid, R.W. (1992). *Staffing of mental health organizations, United States: Selected years from 1955 to 1988.* May, No. 204, p. 16. Mental Health Statistical Note.

Regier, D.A., & Robins, L.N. (1991). Introduction. In D.A. Regier & L.N. Robins (Eds.), *Psychiatric disorders in America: The epidemiologic catchment area study.* (pp. 1-10). New York: The Free Press.

Regier, D.A., Goldberg, I.D., Burns, B.J., Hankin, J., Hoeper, E.W., & Nycz, G.R. (1982). Specialist/generalist division of responsibility for patients with mental disorders. *Archives of General Psychiatry, 39*(2), 219-224.

Regier, D.A., Farmer, M.E., Rae, D.S., Myers, J.K., Kramer, M., Robins, L.N., George, L.K., Karno, M., & Locke, B.Z. (1993). One-month prevalence of mental disorders in the United States and sociodemographic characteristics: The Epidemiologic Catchment Area program. *Acta Psychiatrica Scandinavica, 88*(1), 35-47.

Regier, D.A., Goldberg, I.D., & Taube, C.A. (1978). The de facto U.S. mental health services system: A public health perspective. *Archives of General Psychiatry, 35*(6), 685-693.

Schulberg, H.C., Madonia, M.J., Block, M.R., Coulehan, J.L., Scott, C.P., Rodriguez, E., & Black, A. (1995). Major depression in primary care practice: Clinical characteristics and treatment implications. *Psychosomatics, 36*, 129-137.

Taube, C.A., & Burns, B.J. (1988). Mental health services system research: The National Institute of Mental Health program. *Health Services Research, 22*, 837-855.

Youth Entering
an Emergency Shelter Care Facility:
Prior Involvement in Juvenile Justice
and Mental Health Systems

Alan J. Litrownik
Heather N. Taussig
John A. Landsverk
Ann F. Garland

SUMMARY. Two hundred and ninety five youth between 11 and 17 years of age who entered an emergency shelter care facility reported on their

Alan J. Litrownik and Heather N. Taussig are affiliated with the Center for Research on Child and Adolescent Mental Health Services, SDSU/UCSD Joint Doctoral Program in Clinical Psychology. John A. Landsverk is affiliated with the Center for Research on Child and Adolescent Mental Health Services, School of Social Work, San Diego State University. Ann F. Garland is affiliated with the Center for Research on Child and Adolescent Mental Health Services, Department of Psychiatry, University of California at San Diego.

The authors would like to express their appreciation to the project staff, interviewers, and the staff at the Polinsky Children's Center, San Diego Department of Social Services. A special thanks is extended to the children and youth who made this work possible.

The research reported herein was supported by a grant from the National Institute of Mental Health that established the Center for Research on Child and Adolescent Mental Health Services (Grant No. MH-46078).

Address correspondence to: Alan J. Litrownik, PhD, Center for Research on Child and Adolescent Mental Health Services, 9245 Sky Park Court, Suite 228, San Diego, CA 92123.

[Haworth co-indexing entry note]: "Youth Entering an Emergency Shelter Care Facility: Prior Involvement in Juvenile Justice and Mental Health Systems." Litrownik, Alan J. et al. Co-published simultaneously in *Journal of Social Service Research* (The Haworth Press, Inc.) Vol. 25, No. 3, 1999, pp. 5-19; and: *Mental Health Services and Sectors of Care* (ed: Enola K. Proctor, Nancy Morrow-Howell, and Arlene Stiffman) The Haworth Press, Inc., 1999, pp. 5-19. Single or multiple copies of this article are available for a fee from The Haworth Document Delivery Service [1-800-342-9678, 9:00 a.m. - 5:00 p.m. (EST). E-mail address: getinfo@haworthpressinc.com].

prior involvement with mental health and criminal justice systems. More than a quarter indicated a prior arrest, 10.5% reported a hospital admission, and 43.1% said they had received counseling. An overall logistic regression model revealed that youth who had received counseling prior to entry were almost 3 times more likely to be released to an adult who was not a relative or friend than youth who had not received counseling. Implications for the coordination of services from multiple sectors are discussed. *[Article copies available for a fee from The Haworth Document Delivery Service: 1-800-342-9678. E-mail address: getinfo@haworth pressinc.com]*

KEYWORDS. Mental health services, child welfare system, coordinated services, youth

As evidenced by this volume, there is a growing concern that children and youth who are in need of mental health services not only evidence multiple problems, but also tend to end up being passed from one public service agency to another (e.g., child welfare, juvenile delinquency, mental health). The result is a fragmentation of services, due in part to the lack of an identified unit or agency responsible for coordinating these services (Glisson & James, 1992; Hoagwood, Jensen, Petti, & Burns, 1996).

Much of the research that has responded to this concern has focused on children who enter the child welfare or child protective system. Specifically, investigators have assessed the functioning of children and youth placed in the child welfare system due to maltreatment and documented their need for mental health services (e.g., Halfon, Berkowitz, & Klee, 1992; Hochstadt, Jaudes, Zimo, & Schacter, 1987; Landsverk, Litrownik, Newton, Ganger, & Remmer, 1996; McIntyre & Kessler, 1986; Thompson & Fuhr, 1992). After reviewing these studies, Landsverk (in press) claimed that well over half of the children and youth in the welfare system are in need of mental health services. While some (e.g., Halfon et al., 1992) report that those in need do not always receive necessary services, others (e.g., Garland, Landsverk, Hough, & Ellis-MacLeod, 1996) have found that services are readily provided, especially for older children and youth. In fact, Hoagwood et al. (1996) suggest that many young children who are in need of mental health services are likely to receive services as a result of first being identified by non-mental health systems such as child welfare. Thus, the child welfare system oftentimes functions as the gateway to receipt of mental health services (Landsverk, in press).

Additionally, children and youth entering the child welfare system have been found to be at greater risk for subsequent arrests during adolescence (Widom, 1994). This finding, along with the suggestion that the child welfare system serves as a gateway for mental health services receipt, have led to a number of recent calls to develop and apply appropriate screening assessments for children entering this system (e.g., Boren, Kimmel, Riley, Jordan, Kates, & Morrison, 1996; Kendall, Dale & Plakitsis, 1995; Simmons & Weinman, 1991). The expectation is that early identification of problems in children entering the child protective system can be addressed, thus preventing subsequent problems that would lead to later encounters with other service sectors.

While the empirical literature supports targeting children and youth entering the welfare system, there is a lack of information about whether early involvement in other systems might serve as a gateway into the welfare system. This becomes especially relevant when we consider that the foster care system is already overburdened, and some have claimed that it faces an impending crisis (Rosenfeld, Pilowsky, Fine, Thorpe, Fein, Simms, Halfon, Irwin, Alfaro, Saletsky, & Nickman, 1997). If children and youth entering the welfare system have been previously involved with other systems, then some of the burden placed on the welfare system can be shifted to other systems (e.g., mental health, criminal justice).

A study conducted by our group here in San Diego (Blumberg, Landsverk, Ellis-MacLeod, Ganger, & Culver, 1996) had as its primary objective the description of the overlap between a foster care sample and public mental health service use. While 17.4% ($n = 235$) of the welfare sample ($N = 1,352$) was found to be receiving public mental health services, only 38 (or 16.2%) of those who were receiving these services obtained them prior to entry into out-of-home care. Thus, the only study that has looked at prior multi-system involvement of children and youth entering the welfare system reported little prior involvement with the public mental health system.

Blumberg et al. (1996) did find that the children and youth who were involved in both systems were older and less likely to be placed in kinship care. This later finding has implications for how prior system involvement might be related to the way in which the child protective system handles a new case. That is, prior involvement with the mental health system may lead to the welfare system placing children in more restrictive environments (i.e., with non-kin). This has both legal and psychosocial implications since the federal Adoption and Child Welfare Assistance Act (P.L. 96-272) identifies reunification as the preferred placement option, and many argue that a familiar placement (i.e., with relatives) is desired when out-of-home care is necessary (Bulkley, Feller, Stern, & Roe, 1996). In fact, there is evidence indicating that children and youth in kinship care have fewer behavior problems than those placed with non-relatives (Landsverk, Litrownik, Newton, Ganger, & Remmer, 1996), and those with more behavior problems are also less likely to be reunified with their biological parent(s) (see Landsverk, Davis,

Ganger, Newton, & Johnson, 1996). Thus, if prior system involvement (e.g., mental health, juvenile delinquency) is a result of problem behaviors, then we would expect this involvement to determine, in part, the placement of children and youth within the child protective system.

Emergency shelter care facilities have as their major goal the protection of children and youth who are at risk for being maltreated. Typically, these facilities provide a temporary safe haven while risk is assessed and more permanent living options are identified, including reunification. In order to better serve children and youth, many shelters are now attempting to conduct more thorough assessments of children and youth who enter their doors. If thorough assessment is a goal and it takes longer for those who have more problems, then we might expect longer stays for children and youth who have been previously involved with other systems.

Blumberg et al.'s (1996) finding that children being served by multiple public service sectors were older suggests that any attempt to describe prior system involvement for children entering the child welfare system ought to focus on older children or youth. In fact, prior studies examining multiple system involvement of children in the welfare system have either (1) identified youth who were currently involved with mental health and delinquency systems and determined if there was prior involvement with the child welfare system, or (2) identified children who entered the child welfare system and followed them to see if they became involved in other systems, e.g., arrests (see Widom, 1994). Taking this perspective, it is not unexpected to find investigators concluding that cost-effective interventions can be mounted early on when a child enters the child welfare system, thus preventing subsequent problems that require more restrictive interventions by other systems (e.g., criminal justice, mental health).

Before we limit our focus to only one gateway, i.e., child welfare system, we need to know if youth who are currently entering the welfare system have had prior involvement with other systems. In an effort to respond to this need we collected information about a cohort of youth, 11 to 17 years of age, who entered an emergency shelter care facility in San Diego, California during a 6-month period (April to October, 1995).

The specific objectives of the present study were to: (1) determine the extent of prior service system involvement of youth who were entering the child welfare system (i.e., at the initial point of entry–emergency shelter care facility), (2) identify characteristics of the youth that are related to prior involvement with the mental health and juvenile delinquency systems, and (3) examine the relationship between prior system involvement and outcomes (i.e., length of time in the shelter placement, to whom the youth were released).

METHODS

Subjects

The Polinsky Children's Center, the only emergency shelter care facility for children and youth in the central and southern regions of San Diego County, opened its doors in October of 1994. These regions include large urban areas (e.g., City of San Diego with a population of over 1 million), cities close to the Mexican border, suburbs, and rural mountain towns. This new facility had the capacity to accommodate more children than the previous site and to do so in an environment that is child friendly. In addition, the Department of Social Services saw the opening of the new center as an opportunity to develop and implement protocols for screening all children and youth who entered the facility. As part of the development process, staff from the Center for Research on Child and Adolescent Mental Health Services consulted with Polinsky administrators to determine the objectives of the screening assessments. Following the identification of objectives, potential measures were reviewed, and pilot testing was conducted. The data collected from one of these pilot tests are utilized in the present paper.

Specifically, all youth between the ages of 11 and 17 years of age who entered the emergency shelter care facility between April 18, 1996 and October 11, 1996 were scheduled to complete an intake interview. Of the 466 youth who passed through the Polinsky Center doors, 110 were already active cases that were entering the Polinsky Center as they made the transition from one placement to another. The remaining 356 youth were new entries (i.e., they did not have an open or active case with the San Diego County Department of Social Services). A total of 295 (82.9%) of the new entry youth completed the intake screening interview. Intake interviews were not completed for 61 of the new entry youth (almost half of these youth were Mexican citizens and did not speak English, and the other half were missed primarily due to logistic factors, e.g., late night entry and early morning release before the intake could be completed).

The mean age for the 295 youth was 13.6 years with a standard deviation of 1.7. Additional descriptive information about the youth who completed the intake interview is presented in Table 1. It should also be noted that according to facility records, 26 or 8.8% of the 295 youth had been admitted to the emergency shelter care facility in the previous 6 to 12 months. Though previously admitted to the Polinsky Center, a case had not been formally opened in the child welfare system for these youth.

Procedures

As indicated previously, the pilot screening program for youth was implemented shortly after the new shelter opened. All youth entering the facility

TABLE 1. Sample Characteristics

Sociodemographic Factors and Reason for Entry	Sample (N = 295)	
	n	%
Age (Years)		
11	39	13.2
12	51	17.3
13	54	18.3
14	54	18.3
15	51	17.3
16	32	10.8
17	14	4.7
Gender		
Male	111	37.6
Female	184	62.4
Ethnicity		
Caucasian	133	45.1
African American	71	24.1
Hispanic	65	22.0
Native American	10	3.4
Asian/Pacific Islander	16	5.4
Entry Reason		
Sexual Abuse	32	10.8
Physical Abuse	74	25.1
Neglect	18	.61
Emotional Abuse	13	4.4
Caretaker Absence	146	49.5
Out-of-Town Inquiry	12	4.1

were to be interviewed by an intake worker at the time of entry. Intake workers had participated in the development of the interview, and all had gone through an in-service training prior to implementation of this pilot. During the pilot there were times when the intake staff were not available to complete a youth's interview at entry because of other responsibilities (e.g., responding to crises, supervision of other staff) or they were busy with a number of other entering children and youth. When this occurred youth were checked in and escorted to their living quarters. As soon as possible, usually within a 24-hour period, an intake worker contacted the youth and conducted the interview. These initial intake interviews typically lasted 15 to 20 minutes.

Measures

Intake Interview. The intake interview consisted of a number of questions for youth about their current and past history of risk behaviors (e.g., substance use, suicide ideation and attempts) and consequences or encounters with other systems of care (e.g., counseling, psychiatric hospitalizations, and arrests). If respondents endorsed engaging in these behaviors or experiencing the identified outcomes, follow-up questions asked about when it last occurred, how often and when it first happened or began. These questions, and others (e.g., gang affiliation) asked at intake, were selected in order to provide the staff at the shelter with information about potential problem behaviors that might place the youth or others in the shelter at risk. Additionally, questions about how the youth spent their free time, need for and use of prescription medications, etc., were asked to insure adequate care at the shelter.

Social Service Record Reviews. The San Diego Department of Social Services keeps computerized records for each entry episode. The data for the time period, April 18 to October 11, 1995 (e.g., identification code, date of entry, age, reason for entry, length of stay, release type) were downloaded and merged with data files containing information from the intake assessments. Codes for entry reason (i.e., problem codes) included specific information about perpetrators, as well as additional specification (e.g., parent refuses to care for child, parent unable to care for child because of substance use). These specific codes were collapsed within major categories (e.g., sexual abuse, physical abuse, emotional abuse, neglect, out-of-town inquiry, and caretaker absent/incapacitated). Similarly, information on release type included 40 categories that varied based on whether the youth was released, detained, or placed with a mom, dad, specified relative (e.g., grandmother, female relative, etc.), close friend, or specified stranger (e.g., certified or long-term foster care home, foster care agency, other agency). These categories were collapsed resulting in a dichotomous outcome for release type: (1) released, placed or detained with family or close friends of the family, and (2) released, placed or detained with other non-related adult. It should be noted that 11 youth were not classified on this variable since they did not fit into either of these categories (i.e., 9 had run away from the shelter and their release was coded as AWOL, and 2 had been released in their own custody).

RESULTS

Prior Involvement in Service Sectors

Based on self-reports from youth who were new entries at the emergency shelter care facility run by the San Diego County Department of Social

Services, 25.1% had prior involvement with the criminal justice system (i.e., previously been arrested), and 43.1% and 10.5% had been exposed to the mental health system (i.e., received counseling or been hospitalized in a psychiatric facility, respectively). It is interesting to note (see Table 2) that for those who had received counseling, more than half had received it within the past year, and fully one-quarter were currently receiving services. This same trend was evidenced in those who reported having been admitted to a psychiatric hospital.

Factors Related to Prior System Involvement

The relationships between prior service sector involvement and sociode-mographic factors (i.e., gender, ethnicity, and age) were examined using the chi-square statistic. Gender was not related to any of the three variables indicating prior service sector involvement, while ethnicity was significantly related to receipt of counseling $(\chi^2(4) = 29.19, p < .001)$. This difference appeared to be due to the large percentage of Caucasian and Native American

TABLE 2. Self-Reported Prior System Involvement

Self-Reported Item	Sample (N = 295)	
	n	%
Ever Arrested		
Yes	74	25.1
No	221	74.9
Ever Receive Counseling		
Yes	127	43.1
No	168	56.9
When Receive Counseling		
In last week	29	26.2
In last 6 months	18	16.2
In last year	11	9.8
More than year ago	53	47.8
Admitted to Psychiatric Hospital		
Yes	31	10.5
No	264	89.5
When Admitted to Psychiatric Hospital		
In last year	15	57.7
Over year ago	11	42.3

youth who had received counseling (77 of 133, and 5 of 10, respectively) as compared to those who were African-American (28 of 71), Hispanic (15 of 65), and Asian/Pacific Islander (2 of 16). Though age was not related to psychiatric hospitalization, there was a significant linear relationship (i.e., Mantel-Haenszel test for linear association) between age and arrests $(\chi^2(1) =$ 8.86, $p < .01$) and receipt of counseling $(\chi^2(1) = 5.08, p < .05)$, suggesting that the older the youth got, the more likely they were to receive counseling as well as to be arrested.

Relationship of Prior Sector Involvement to Outcomes

The two variables of interest in terms of outcomes of the current episode of care within the emergency shelter care facility were (1) length of stay (days), and (2) release type (family or close family friend versus non-related adult). Youth stayed at the Polinsky Center between 1 and 56 days with a mean of 3.6 days (standard deviation = 4.7). Nearly half (i.e., 49.5%) were released within 2 days, and only 5.1% remained for more than 7 days. A total of 217 (or 76.4%) of the youth were released to their parent(s), relative, or close family friend.

In an effort to begin to understand how prior service sector involvement may be related to the handling of a case within the child welfare system, we looked at the relationship between reports of prior arrests, counseling and psychiatric hospitalization, and length of stay in the shelter as well as the type of release. Summary bivariate analyses for the two outcomes (i.e., type of release and length of stay) and the three indicators of prior sector involvement are presented in Tables 3 and 4. As indicated in Table 3, length of stay at the shelter was not related to any of the three indicators of prior service sector involvement.

On the other hand, both of the indicators of prior involvement in the mental health system (i.e., counseling and psychiatric hospitalization) were significantly related to release type $(\chi^2(1) = 10.0, p < .01;$ and $\chi^2(1) = 5.01,$ $p < .05$, respectively). Specifically, those youth who had prior involvement in the mental health system, either through counseling or psychiatric hospitalization, were approximately 2.4 times more likely to be released to a stranger (i.e., adult who was not a relative or close family friend) than those who did not have any prior involvement. Involvement in the criminal justice system through a prior arrest was not related to release type.

In order to separate the contribution of various predictive factors on release type, an overall logistic regression model was evaluated. Sociodemographic and reason for entry factors were entered in the first two blocks of the regression analysis, with the three indicators of prior service system involvement entered in the third and final block. For the categorical factor of ethnicity, all groups were compared to the Caucasian group, and for entry reason, all

TABLE 3. Days at Polinsky Center as a Function of Prior Service System Involvement

Item	n	Mean	sd	p value
Ever Been Arrested				
No	221	3.60	4.87	.795
Yes	74	3.43	4.18	
Ever Received Outpatient Counseling				
No	168	3.20	2.60	.174
Yes	127	4.03	6.50	
Ever Admitted to Psychiatric Hospital				
No	264	3.63	4.93	.439
Yes	31	2.94	1.83	

p values are based on t-tests for independent samples with adjustments for unequal variances when appropriate (e.g., ever received outpatient counseling).

TABLE 4. Relationship Between Self-Reported System Involvement and Release Type

Determinant	Relative Risk	95% Confidence Interval	Probability
Previously Arrested	1.394	(0.7494; 2.5919)	.29
Received Counseling	2.439	(1.3932; 4.2699)	.002
Admitted to Psychiatric Hospital	2.412	(1.0957; 5.3101)	.025

2×2 chi-square analyses (i.e., Relative Risk) were conducted on 284 cases examining the relationship between each of the predictors with the outcome of release type (family or close friend vs. other) independently.

groups were compared to the Caretaker Absent/Incapacitated group. The overall model, presented in Table 5, was significant ($\chi^2(3) = 12.4, p < .01$). While ethnicity was not a significant predictor overall, the Native American youth were 4.5 times more likely ($p < .05$) to be placed with a stranger than Caucasian youth. Entry reason was significant, due to the fact that youth who

TABLE 5. Standard Logistic Regression Identifying Predictors of Release Type

Determinant	b	Odds Ratio	95% C.I.	Significance (*p* <)
Native American	1.51	4.53	(1.31; 15.74)	.05
Sexual Abuse	.94	2.57	(1.11; 5.93)	.05
Physical Abuse	− .89	.41	(.18; .96)	.05
Counseling	1.02	2.77	(1.41; 5.46)	.01

Dependent Variable = Type of Release (Relative or close friend versus Stranger). Nonsignificant Independent Variables: Gender, Age, African-American, Hispanic, Asian/Pacific Islander, Neglect, Emotional Abuse, Out-of-Town Inquiry, Ever Arrested, and Ever Hospitalized

were sexually abused were 2.5 times more likely to be placed with a stranger, and youth who were physically abused were approximately 2.5 times more likely to be placed with a relative or friend, than the youth who entered because of an absent or incapacitated caretaker. Finally, youth who had reported prior involvement with the mental health service system through counseling were almost 2.8 times as likely (*p* < .05) to be placed with a stranger than those who had not reported prior counseling experience.

DISCUSSION

In summary, youth entering an emergency shelter care facility indicate that they have had extensive involvement with other service systems. This involvement was related to the youth's ethnicity (i.e., Caucasian and Native American youth were more likely to have received counseling), and to their age (i.e., the older the youth the more likely they had received prior counseling and been arrested). Finally, youth who had received prior counseling were almost three times as likely to be released to a stranger when they left the shelter than those who had not.

Prior studies examining multi-system involvement have typically targeted children in the child protective system and observed to see if they then received subsequent needed mental health services (e.g., Blumberg et al., 1996), or entered the criminal justice system at some later point in time (e.g., Widom, 1994). Such a focus predisposes investigators to discover that child welfare involvement leads to involvement in other systems (e.g., serving as a gateway for mental health services, and placing children at risk for entering the criminal justice system). In the present study we identified an older cohort of youth entering the child protective system, and asked for retrospective information about prior experiences with mental health and criminal justice systems. While suffering from all of the limitations of any retrospective study, the current results do suggest that the relationship between child welfare involvement and involvement in the mental health and criminal justice systems is not unidirectional. In fact, it appears that early involvement in any of these systems of care may place an individual at risk for later involvement in the other systems.

More than half of the children and youth in foster care have been identified as needing mental health services (see Halfon et al., 1992; Hochstadt et al., 1987; Landsverk, in press; McIntyre & Kessler, 1986). Though the current cohort of youth were not as embedded within the welfare system as those in out-of-home care, 40% did indicate that they had already been exposed to counseling. If these self-reports of prior system involvement reflect actual experiences of youth at the beginning point of entry into the welfare system, then it is already the case that youth with multiple problems are being presented to the child welfare system. And, if recent changes in social policy will likely lead to a dumping of even more children and youth from other systems into the child protective system as Rosenfeld et al. (1997) warn, then the time to heed the call to coordinate services (Glisson & James, 1992; Hoagwood et al., 1997) is now.

There is a literature (see Landsverk, in press; Widom, 1994) pointing to the need to make sure that children and youth in the child protective system receive appropriate mental health services. Coordination of such services has the potential to reduce the risk of more serious subsequent mental health problems as well as reduce the risk of involvement in the criminal justice system. While such coordination is still lacking, it is the case that many of the children and youth within the child welfare system do receive mental health services (e.g., Blumberg et al., 1996; Garland et al., 1996; Halfon & Klee, 1992). The results of the present study suggest that many of the youth who enter the child protective system have already received mental health services (e.g., counseling), and for most, these services were provided within a year of this entry. If these mental health services were effective we might expect that they could prevent subsequent involvement in the child welfare system for some children and youth. More specifically, just as the child welfare system serves as a gateway for needed mental health services that can prevent subsequent problems, it would be appropriate for the mental health system to serve as the gateway for appropriate child welfare or social services.

The emergency shelter care facility in San Diego County serves as the initial point of entry into the child welfare system. While housed in this facility, decisions about each youth's further involvement in the system are made including where they will be housed subsequently. The results of the present study indicate that youth with prior involvement in the mental health system are treated differently. That is, they are less likely to be reunified or released to a familiar caretaker (i.e., parent, relative, or close family friend) thus necessitating the expenditure of additional child welfare resources. This finding is consistent with empirical studies that report children and youth in foster care are less likely to be reunified with their parents as well as less likely to be placed with relatives if they evidence more behavior problems (Landsverk, Davis, Ganger, Newton, & Johnson, 1996; Landsverk, Litrownik, Newton, Ganger, & Remmer, 1996).

While a number of studies suggest that stability of a foster placement is related to problem behaviors (see Palmer, 1996), we did not find that length of stay at the shelter care facility was impacted by prior system involvement. This may not be unexpected given that the objective of an emergency shelter is not stable placement in the facility, but rather interim protection. On the other hand, the newly opened Polinsky Center had as one of its objectives, the assessment of children and youth so the next placement would be the most appropriate one. With this objective we might expect that those youth with more problems would need more thorough assessments before they were placed (i.e., released). The failure to find a relationship between prior system involvement (and assumed behavior problems) and days at the facility can be accounted for, in part, by the fact that almost half of the youth were released within 2 days (i.e., a decision was made not to move the case further into the system). This initial decision would likely mask any impact of prior system involvement on length of stay.

METHODOLOGICAL ISSUES
AND LIMITATIONS OF THE STUDY

The present study is viewed as the first step in expanding our perspective on how children and youth move between the child welfare system and other public systems of care. While the results indicate future examination of the movement between systems is warranted, there are some limitations to the current findings. First, we recognize that the present results are based on retrospective self-reports of youth who entered a specific child welfare system (i.e., San Diego County). Admittedly, we must be cautious in relying on these retrospective self-reports as their reliability and validity have not been established. It is also the case that the specific findings may be a function of the structure and operation of the child welfare system in San Diego County. For example, not all protective service agencies utilize a single point of entry (i.e., emergency shelter care facility). Thus, the generalizability of the current results to other child welfare systems must await additional study.

DIRECTIONS FOR FUTURE STUDY

Nevertheless, the results of the present study indicate that many youth entering the child welfare system may have prior involvement with the mental health and criminal justice systems, and that this prior involvement can lead to how the welfare system responds to the case. Our traditional unidirectional approach to understanding multi-system involvement needs to be expanded, as well as our recommendations for how services can best be provided. Specifically, prospective studies that follow children and youth as they move from one system to another will provide us with a better understanding of the pathways to involvement in public service sectors. Finally, we need to develop and evaluate the efficacy (as well as effectiveness) of interventions that prevent the dumping of problem children and youth into the child welfare system.

REFERENCES

Blumberg, E., Landsverk, J., Ellis-MacLeod, E., Ganger, W., & Culver, S. (1996). Use of the public mental health system by children in foster care: Client characteristics and service use patterns. *Journal of Mental Health Administration, 23,* 389-405.

Boren, S. I., Kimmel, H., Riley, A., Jordan, K. M., Kates, W., & Morrison, J. (February, 1996). *Mental health screening of children at entry to foster care.* Paper presented at the Ninth Annual Research Conference, A System of Care for Children's Mental Health, Tampa, Florida.

Bulkley, J. A., Feller, J. N., Stern, P., & Roe, R. (1996). Child abuse and neglect laws and legal proceedings. In J. Briere, L. Berliner, J.A. Bulkley, C. Jenny, & T. Reid (Eds.) *The APSAC Handbook on Child Maltreatment.* Thousand Oaks: Sage, pp. 271-296.

Garland, A. F., Landsverk, J. L., Hough, R. L., & Ellis-MacLeod, E. (1996). Type of maltreatment as a predictor of mental health service use for children in foster care. *Child Abuse & Neglect, 20,* 675-688.

Glisson, C., & James, L. (1992). The interorganizational coordination of services to children in state custody. *Administration in Social Work, 16,* 65-80.

Halfon, N., Berkowitz, G., & Klee, L. (1992). Mental health service utilization by children in foster care in California. *Pediatrics, 89,* 1238-1244.

Hoagwood, K., Jensen, P. S., Petti, T., & Burns, B. J. (1996). Outcome of mental health care for children and adolescents: I. A comprehensive conceptual model. *Journal of the American Academy of Child and Adolescent Psychiatry, 35,* 1055-1063.

Hochstadt, N. J., Jaudes, P. K., Zimo, D. A., & Schacter, J. (1987). The medical and psychosocial needs of children entering foster care. *Child Abuse & Neglect, 11*, 53-62.

Kendall, J., Dale, G., & Plakitsis, S. (1995). The mental health needs of children entering the child welfare system: A guide for case workers. *The APSAC Advisor, 8*, 10-13.

Landsverk, J. (in press). Foster care and pathways in mental health services. In P. Curtis and G. Dale (Eds.) *The Foster Care Crisis: Translating Research into Practice and Policy.* The University of Nebraska Press.

Landsverk, J., Davis, I., Ganger, W., Newton, R., & Johnson, I. (1996). Impact of child psychosocial functioning on reunification from out-of-home care. *Children and Youth Services Review, 18*, 447-462.

Landsverk, J., Litrownik, A., Newton, R., Ganger, W., & Remmer, J. (1996). *Psychological Impact of Child Maltreatment.* Final Report to National Center on Child Abuse and Neglect.

McIntyre, A., & Kessler, T. (1986). Psychological disorders among foster children. *Journal of Clinical Child Psychology, 15*, 297-303.

Palmer, S. E. (1996). Placement stability and inclusive practice in foster care: An empirical study. *Children and Youth Services Review, 18*, 589-601.

Rosenfeld, A. A., Pilowsky, D. J., Fine, P., Thorpe, M., Fein, E., Simms, M. D., Halfon, N., Irwin, M., Alfaro, J., Saletsky, R. & Nickman, S. (1997). Foster care: An update. *Journal of the American Academy of Child & Adolescent Psychiatry, 36*, 448-457.

Simmons, J. T., & Weinman, M. L. (1991). Self-esteem, adjustment, and locus of control among youth in an emergency shelter. *Journal of Community Psychology, 19*, 277-280.

Thompson, A. H., & Fuhr, D. (1992). Emotional disturbance in 50 children in the care of a child welfare system. *Journal of Social Service Research, 15*, 95-112.

Widom, C. S. (1994). Childhood victimization and adolescent problem behaviors. In R. D. Ketterlinus & M. E. Lamb (Eds.) *Adolescent problem behaviors: Issues and research.* New Jersey: Erlbaum, pp. 127-164.

Physician-Patient Gender and the Recognition and Treatment of Depression in Primary Care

Lee W. Badger
Michael Berbaum
Patricia A. Carney
Allen J. Dietrich
Mary Owen
John T. Stem

SUMMARY. This study investigates the relationships among patient's gender, physician's gender, and physician's inquiries about depression symptoms and psychosocial stressors, treatment and subsequent medi-

Lee W. Badger is affiliated with the Graduate School of Social Service at Fordham University. Michael Berbaum is affiliated with the Institute for Social Science Research, The University of Alabama. Patricia A. Carney is affiliated with the Department of Family and Community Medicine, Dartmouth Medical School. Allen J. Dietrich is affiliated with the Department of Community and Family Medicine, Dartmouth Medical School. Mary Owen is affiliated with the Department of Medical Education, University of Washington. John T. Stem is affiliated with the Institute for Social Science Research, University of Alabama.

The authors thank Carolyn Neiswender, Marian Swindell and Ali Winters at the University of Alabama, M. Scottie Eliassen at Dartmouth, and Jenny Struijk at the University of Washington for their assistance throughout the conduct of this study.

This study was funded by a grant from the John D. and Catherine T. MacArthur Foundation.

A portion of this paper was presented at the International Conference on Mental Health Problems in the General Health Care Sector, NIMH, September 1997.

[Haworth co-indexing entry note]: "Physician-Patient Gender and the Recognition and Treatment of Depression in Primary Care." Badger, Lee W. et al. Co-published simultaneously in *Journal of Social Service Research* (The Haworth Press, Inc.) Vol. 25, No. 3, 1999, pp. 21-39; and: *Mental Health Services and Sectors of Care* (ed: Enola K. Proctor, Nancy Morrow-Howell, and Arlene Stiffman) The Haworth Press, Inc., 1999, pp. 21-39. Single or multiple copies of this article are available for a fee from The Haworth Document Delivery Service [1-800-342-9678, 9:00 a.m. - 5:00 p.m. (EST). E-mail address: getinfo@haworthpressinc.com].

21

cal record notation of depression in primary care. One hundred forty-six physicians at three sites were visited twice by a standardized patient (SP) who enacted either major depression with a psychosocial presentation or minor depression with a somatic presentation. Each of the two cases was portrayed by both male and female SPs who were assigned randomly to physicians. Results showed high rates of inquiry about depression symptoms and treatment, but rates varied considerably by presentation and across physician-patient gender combinations. Male physicians explored symptoms and discussed a diagnosis with female patients significantly more often than with male patients. Both male and female physicians recommended counseling more often for patients with the somatic presentation when they were female than when they were male. Record notations followed the same gender pattern. *[Article copies available for a fee from The Haworth Document Delivery Service: 1-800-342-9678. E-mail address: getinfo@haworthpressinc.com]*

KEYWORDS. Depression, gender, primary care, recognition, diagnosis

Primary care clinicians, educators, and policy makers agree that communication about the psychosocial dimension of patients' health is essential to the effective practice of primary care medicine (Ashworth, Williamson & Montano, 1984; Campbell, Neikirk & Hosokawa, 1990; Goldberg, Steele, Johnson & Smith, 1982; Novack, Goldberg, Rowland-Morin, Landau & Wartman, 1989; Schulberg, McClelland & Coulehan, 1986; Schulberg & McClelland, 1987). In spite of this, research about primary care physicians' approaches to the exploration of psychosocial and emotional problems such as major depression is scarce (Burns & Burke, 1985; Schulberg et al., 1986). As many as half of patients with depression may go unrecognized by physicians (Badger et al., 1994; Katon, Berg, Robins et al., 1986; Katon, Kleinman & Rosen, 1982; Katon & Schulberg, 1992) despite its being among the most frequent and treatable disorders in primary care (Hoeper, Nycz, Cleary et al., 1979; Katon, Kleinman & Rosen, 1982; Schulberg et al., 1985). It is suggested that investigation into the influence of physician and patient genders on the conduct of the medical encounter may contribute to a better understanding of the recognition of depression in primary care.

Differential treatment of male and female patients has long been a concern of clinicians and researchers interested in social bias in medical care (Safran, Rogers, Tarlov, McHorney & Ware, 1997; Verbrugge, 1984; Kerssens, 1997 #296). Even though a fundamental assumption of the medical model is that medical care is based on scientific knowledge free from personal norms and values (Kerssens, Bensing & Andela, 1997), there is conjecture that both physician gender and patient gender may nonetheless exert a subtle yet consequential effect (Weisman & Teitelbaum, 1985). The purpose of this study was to investigate the possible effects of physician-patient gender combinations on physicians' inquiries about depression symptoms and subsequent recommendations for treatment.

Studies of physician and patient gender, and their combinations, have yet to provide a clear picture of their impact on medical care. With respect to physician-patient verbal and nonverbal communication in general, for example, several studies have reported that female physicians both conduct longer interviews and talk more extensively about psychosocial issues than do male physicians (Bernzweig, Takayama, Phibbs, Lewis & Pantell, 1997; Hall, Irish, Roter et al., 1994a; Hall, Irish, Roter et al., 1994b; Roter, Lipkin & Korsgard, 1991), yet Weisman and Teitelbaum (1985) found that same sex physician-patient interactions were characterized by more effective communication and stronger rapport than opposite-sex interactions. With respect to postulating etiology or "recognizing" mental disorder, both patient and physician gender appear to exert an influence, although the direction is not clear. For example, Wallen and colleagues (1979) reported that female patients were more likely to have their illnesses attributed to psychological causes when the physician was male but, more recently, Linzer and colleagues (1996) noted that female patients had their symptoms attributed to mental disorder, that is, their mental disorder was "recognized," equally often by male and female physicians. However, male patients were significantly more likely to have symptoms attributed to mental disorder when the physician was female. Yet another study conducted by Simon et al. (1995) found no significant relationship between recognition of depression and patient gender.

There is no greater clarity among reported findings with regard to the effects of physician and patient gender on medical care subsequent to recognition. While several studies have found that female patients receive more of a given service (Verbrugge, 1984), have their activities restricted more often (Safran et al., 1997), and are more likely than male patients to receive a prescription for an antidepressant (Williams et al., 1995), in an epidemiologic survey of over 1900 patients, Simon et al. (1995) reported no gender differences in the likelihood of receiving treatment.

However provocative, prior studies of physician-patient dyads have been criticized both for a failure to control for patient presentation and health status as well as for a failure to randomize assignment of patients to physicians (Bertakis, Helms, Callahan, Azari & Robbins, 1995; Weisman & Teitelbaum, 1985). The purpose of this study, therefore, was to investigate the effect of physician-patient gender combinations on physicians' inquiries about depression symptoms and subsequent treatment with patient presentation controlled using male and female standardized patients (SPs) randomly assigned to physicians. In addition, the literature indicates that primary care patients with mood and anxiety disorders frequently present with vague, somatic symptoms such as headache, abdominal pain, low back pain, dizziness or nervousness (Barrett, Barrett, Oxman & Gerber, 1988; Mathew, Weinman & Mirabi, 1981). In fact, in a study by Kirmayer and colleagues (1993), the psychiatric condition of patients who made somatized presentations was only one-tenth to one-third as likely to be recognized as that of patients who made psychosocial presentations. The tendency of physicians to attend preferentially only to the somatic symptoms, perhaps without a full awareness of the potential underlying psychosocial influences on the patients' illnesses, may be a key factor in the problem of under-recognition (Baughman, 1994). For this reason, the current study was designed to compare two patient presentations of depression, one somatic and one psychosocial. It has been suggested also that primary care physicians have inadequate time to gather information sufficient to make a depression diagnosis (Eisenberg, 1992) and therefore frequently defer mental diagnoses to subsequent visits (Bertakis et al., 1995; Froom, 1988; Pardes, 1979). To study this issue, our research design included both a first assessment and a follow-up interview. We hypothesized that interviews would be longer and recognition and treatment would occur both sooner and more frequently for the psychosocial presentation of major depression than for the somatic presentation of minor depression; both male and female physicians would explore and treat depression more frequently with female patients than male patients; and that female physicians would conduct longer interviews than male physicians regardless of the type of patient presentation.

METHODS

Sample of Physicians

The study took place in three regions close to the research team members (Northern New England, Washington State, Alabama). General internists and family physicians were recruited in the following manner in each region: in Northern New England, through the Dartmouth Co-op, an electronically networked organization of regional physicians; in Washington State, by a member of the medical school faculty from a list of regional members of the family medicine and internal medicine associations; and in Alabama, by the past presidents of the Alabama Association of Family Physicians and the Alabama Association of General Internists from directories of regional members. In each region, initial invitations to participate were extended in mass mailings or electronically; physicians either elected to volunteer or did not respond. Interested physicians were eligible for participation when, by self-report, they met the following criteria: had their practices open to new patients, spent over 50% of their practice time in general medicine (not subspecialty care), and had been practicing at the current location for at least two years. The final sample included 146 physicians. Although we sought to recruit an equivalent number of male and female volunteers, we did not find in either the Alabama or Northern New England regions sufficient numbers of female physicians who practiced full-time and had practices open to new patients. Thus, male physicians predominated in the study sample (n = 97, 66%). Seventy-five physicians were visited by one case, and 71 were visited by the other case. Physician and practice characteristics are shown in Tables 1 and 2.

Physicians were unaware of the mental health focus of the study. Physicians were told in advance that they would be visited twice by the same standardized patient, who would (1) not identify himself or herself as such, (2) portray a case typical in primary care practice, and (3) carry a hidden audio recorder.

Procedure and Data Collection

Two standardized patient (SP) cases were developed to meet DSM-III-R criteria for minor depression and major depression. In the primary care set-

TABLE 1. Crosstabulation of Physician Specialty, Practice Type, and Site by Physician Gender

Physician/Practice Characteristic		Physician Gender					
		Male		Female		Total	
		n	%	n	%	N	%
All Physicians		97	66%	49	34%	146	100%
Research Site							
	New Hampshire	52	36%	17	12%	69	48%
	Washington	22	15%	24	16%	46	31%
	Alabama	23	16%	8	5%	31	21%
Specialty							
	Family Practice	44	30%	30	21%	74	51%
	Internal Medicine	53	36%	19	13%	72	49%
Practice Type							
	Solo Practice	29	20%	6	4%	35	24%
	Group Practice	68	47%	43	29%	111	76%

TABLE 2. Physician and Practice Characteristics by Physician Gender

| | Physician Gender | | | | | |
| Characteristic | Male (n = 97) | | Female (n = 49) | | Whole Sample (N = 146) | |
	Mean	SD	Mean	SD	Mean	SD
Physician						
Age (years)	44.6	7.9	39.6	5.7	42.9	7.6
Years Since Graduation	19.0	8.7	11.8	4.4	16.1	8.4
Years at Current Practice	11.8	9.1	5.8	4.6	9.9	8.4
Adults Seen per Week	92.8	37.4	64.5	27.5	84.2	37.0
Practice						
Percent HMO patients	20.8	16.9	22.1	15.4	21.2	16.4
Percents Medicaid patients	11.7	9.3	17.3	14.5	13.4	11.4
Percent Medicare patients	30.6	16.9	20.9	15.6	27.5	17.1
Percent Private patients	21.4	14.9	21.1	15.2	21.3	14.9
Percent Non-Insured patients	7.8	6.3	12.4	12.3	9.2	8.8

ting patients with mood and anxiety disorders typically present with somatic symptoms. Therefore the first case was a 26-year-old data entry clerk who presented with headaches. S/he also met DSM criteria for minor depression (anhedonia, weight and appetite gain, hypersomnia) and had experienced recent stressful life events (e.g., a divorce, move to the area, and only temporary employment). Since we were interested in treatment of depression as well as its recognition, we also developed a case with a strong likelihood of being immediately recognized and treated. This second case was a 45-year-old corporate loan officer who presented with an inability to concentrate, as well as insomnia, both of which are criterion symptoms of depression. S/he met symptom criteria for major depression (insomnia, inability to concentrate, weight and appetite loss, hopelessness, and depressed mood) and had also experienced recent stressful life events (recent move and separation from family, undesired job change and poor job performance report). Thus, we developed a minor depression case with a somatic presentation and a major depression case with a psychosocial presentation.

At each research site, four males and four females were recruited to serve as SPs. One half of these were assigned to enact the minor depression/somatic case (2 males, 2 females) and the other half were assigned to enact the major depression/psychosocial presentation (2 males, 2 females). Case development, testing, and training tapes were prepared at the Northern New England site and shared among the other sites so as to enhance intra-performance and inter-performance reliabilities of SPs. SPs assigned to each patient case were coached, both individually and together, regarding behavior, affect, and scripted responses. At the first visit, each SP had a scripted and fixed "presenting complaint"–headaches for the minor depression case and inability to concentrate and insomnia for the major depression case–and, at the second visit, reported feeling "about 50% better, but still not like my old self." Thereafter, coaching was focused on maintaining a "natural" dialogue with the physician and limiting the number of symptoms and other information that could be volunteered by the SP. Additional scripted information could, however, be elicited by physicians' inquiries. Approximately three to five hours of active coaching per SP were necessary in order to achieve accurate and consistent performance. Prior to making study visits each SP was interviewed and critiqued by five primary care physicians, usually members of the local medical school faculty who were unaware of the study purposes. SPs were considered ready to go into the field when their combined intra-performance consistency and accuracy in using the Encounter Rating Form (described below) was greater than 90%. The consistency and accuracy of SPs' performances were monitored by audio tape.

SPs were randomly assigned to physicians. Each SP made his or her appointments, paid for the visits in cash, and asked to defer any laboratory work until their medical insurance "kicked in." The same SP made both visits to the given physician. SPs were obviously aware that the study concerned depression, although they were unaware of specific hypotheses. SPs knew that there were male and female SPs and may, therefore, have speculated that gender was a hypothesis.

Measures

Immediately following each of the two visits, SPs completed an Encounter Rating Form, a structured checklist, which captured the content and length of the medical interview. SPs utilized the audio tape recording of the medical visit while completing these forms. Site coordinators also periodically checked the accuracy of SP checklists against the audio taped medical encounters to ensure accuracy. Two weeks following the second (and last) visit, site coordinators conducted a semi-structured telephone debriefing with participating physicians in order to explore their clinical impressions and diagnostic and treatment reasoning. After completion of all study visits, and after the debriefing call, each SP's medical records were obtained and coded.

Prior investigations of physician recognition, which have typically relied upon medical record notations alone, have been criticized for confounding recognition and record-keeping practices (Burnum, 1989; Robbins, Kirmayer, Cathebras, Yaffe & Dworkind, 1994). Therefore, we chose to broaden our definition of "recognition" to also take into account physician exploration and discussion of depression in addition to chart notation. As shown in the description of our measures in Table 3, we have defined the medical encounter as having four pertinent and interrelated activities: (1) exploration of depression symptoms and associated psychosocial stressors; (2) discussion with the patient of the implications of a depression diagnosis, which we measured in two ways: whether a depression diagnosis was discussed (a dichotomous variable) and, to indicate thoroughness, a count of how many of the relevant topics (etiology, course, prognosis, treatment options, and provision of written material) were discussed; (3) decisions about treatment and follow-up; and (4) notation of depression in the medical chart. We discuss results for each activity in turn.

TABLE 3. Measures of Physician Actions During Medical Interview

Actions	Indices	Possible Range
1. Exploration of:		
Depression	Depressed mood, Anhedonia, Fatigue or loss of energy, Sleep difficulty, Psychomotor retardation or agitation, Sense of worthlessness, Increase or decrease in appetite, Thoughts of death.*	0-8
Psychosocial Stressors	Irritability, Loneliness, Occupation, Recent move, Home situation, Recent divorce, Socail activities, Alcohol and drug use.	0-8
2. Discussion of Implications of Depression Diagnosis	Possibility of depression causing symptoms, Etiology, Prognosis, Possible treatment options, Written material.	0-5
3. Treatment	Prescribe antidepressant medication?	yes, no
	Discuss referral for ongoing counseling?	yes, no
4. Chart Notation	Any mention of depression in the medical chart?	yes, no

*Insomnia was a portion of the standardized presenting complaint. Hence, further investigation into the nature of the sleep difficulty was required. Inability to concentrate was inadvertently omitted from the somatic presentation Encounter Rating Form and therefore was not included for either case in the analysis.

Methods of Analysis

The design of this study involves between-subjects factors (physician gender [M, F]), patient gender [M,F], and case presentation/severity [minor depression/somatic presentation, major depression/psychosocial presentation), as well as the within-subjects factor Visit (visit 1, visit 2). For continuous dependent variables, the analysis of variance for repeated measures was employed. For discrete dependent variables (loglinear) contingency table analysis was employed. The same four factors were included in all analysis. Since the design is a 2 × 2 × 2 × 2, all main effects and interaction tests involved a single numerator degree of freedom and post hoc tests were superfluous. When interactions proved significant, their interpretation superceded discussion of main effects (Kirk, 1995), and hence they are presented first in the tables; however, significant main effects are also noted. To simplify tables, only those interactions that proved significant are listed.

RESULTS

Exploration of Depression Symptoms and Psychosocial Stressors

Across the two visits, physicians elicited an average of 3.8 depression symptoms. Analysis of variance of the number of depression symptoms yielded a Presentation by Visit interaction ($F_{(1,135)}$ = 27.04, p < .001). Neither Physician Gender nor Patient Gender were statistically significant. At Visit 1, physicians elicited a higher number of depression symptoms from SPs with the psychosocial presentation of major depression than they did from SPs with the somatic presentation of minor depression (4.2 vs 2.1). However, at Visit 2 the number of symptoms elicited was not much higher (1.8 vs 1.0). Basically, the more straightforward psychosocial presentation, and more severe symptomatic case of depression, drew physicians' attention about the possibility of depression right away.

Analysis of variance of the number of questions about psychosocial stressors (possible range = 0-8) produced a Physician Gender by Visit interaction ($F_{(1,129)}$ = 4.11, p < .05). Patient Gender was not significant. Physicians asked a greater number of psychosocial questions during Visit 1 than during Visit 2 (3.2 vs. 1.2). Male and female physicians asked similar numbers of questions during Visit 1 (3.1 vs. 3.3), but male physicians asked more questions than female physicians during Visit 2 (1.3 vs .9). Physicians, especially female physicians, appeared to assign investigation of psychosocial stressors to the initial visit, but overall the number of psychosocial inquiries by both male and female physicians was low at both visits.

We wanted to investigate whether the type of patient presentation and gender of either physician or patient were related to the length of time spent with patients, i.e., the duration of the two medical interviews. An analysis of variance yielded several main and two-way interactions as well as a significant four-way interaction among Physician Gender, Patient Gender, Presentation, and Visit (see Table 4). Contrary to expectation, female physicians conducted substantially longer interviews only with male patients portraying the major depression/psychosocial presentation at the initial visit. This was the source of the four-way interaction, shown in the lower-right 2 × 2 corner of Table 5. As expected, somewhat longer interviews were conducted with the major depression/psychosocial case than the minor depression/somatic case.

Discussion with Patient About the Implications of a Depression Diagnosis

Measuring discussion of depression by whether or not the physician had suggested the possibility of depression as a diagnosis (a dichotomous variable), contingency table analysis showed that, by the end of the second visit, significantly more physicians had discussed depression with the major depression/psychosocial case than with the minor depression/somatic case (96% vs. 70%; $\chi^2_{(1)}$ = 3.7, p < .05). Male physicians discussed depression

TABLE 4. Analysis of Variance of Length of Interview by Physician Gender, Patient Gender, Presentation, and Visit

Source of Variation	df	MS[a]	F
Significant Interactions[b]			
Presentation × Visit	1	632.8	14.31*
Physician Gender × Presentation × Visit	1	187.4	4.23*
Physician Gender × Patient Gender × Presentation × Visit	1	250.2	5.65*
Main Effects			
Physician Gender	1	.02	.98
Patient Gender	1	6.3	.06
Presentation (somatic, psychosocial)	1	528.8	4.65*
Visit (1,2)	1	5890.8	133.10*
Error	127	113.8	

*p < .05
[a]Since all terms have one degree of freedom, SS may be omitted (same as MS).
[b]No other interactions reached significance at the α = .05 level. All main effects and interactions were included in the reported model. Interpretation of interactions supersedes interpretation of main effects. Means are shown in Table 5.

TABLE 5. Mean Length of Interview (in minutes) by Physician Gender, Patient Gender, Presentation, and Visit*

Physican Gender	Case			
Patient Gender	Minor Depression/Somatic		Major Depression/Psychosocial	
	Visit 1	Visit 2	Visit 1	Visit 2
Male Physicians				
Male Patients	18.5	13.0	24.8	11.5
Female Patients	20.2	15.9	24.9	11.9
Female Physicians				
Male Patients	19.6	12.4	31.0	11.2
Female Patients	19.6	9.6	21.1	15.1

*This four-way interaction (Physician Gender × Patient Gender × Presentation × Visit) was significant ($F_{(1,127)}$ = 5.65, p < .05; see Table 4)

with 39% of male and 92% of female patients with the minor depression/somatic presentation ($\chi^2_{(1)}$ = 14.4, p < .001), whereas female physicians discussed depression equivalently often with both genders (73% vs. 68%).

Using the second approach to measure the thoroughness of discussion, namely a count of how many of the relevant topics (etiology, course, prognosis, treatment options, and provision of written material) were discussed, analysis of variance revealed several significant two-way interactions, as shown in Table 6. However, the significant three-way interaction among Physician Gender, Patient Gender, and Visit ($F_{(1,130)}$ = 9.13, p < .05) supersedes interpretation of several of the two-way interactions. Female physicians discussed depression more thoroughly with female patients during the initial (2.4 vs. 2.1) encounter and with male patients during the second encounter (1.4 vs. .9). At the first encounter, male physicians engaged in less discussion than female physicians, although they discussed depression equivalently with both male and female patients (1.5 vs. 1.6). They exhibited behavior similar to that of female physicians during the second encounter by also discussing depression more frequently with male patients (2.0 vs. .9).

Decisions About Treatment

Decisions about treatment were assessed by noting whether physicians suggested antidepressant drug therapy and/or recommended counseling, or both. Overwhelmingly, SPs with the major depression/psychosocial presentation were offered antidepressant prescriptions more often than SPs with the

TABLE 6. Thoroughness of Discussion of the Implications of Depression as a Diagnosis

Source of Variation	df	MS[a]	F
Significant Interactions[b]			
Physician Gender × Patient Gender × Presentation × Visit	1	11.66	9.13*
Physician Gender × Patient Gender	1	8.06	4.22*
Physician Gender × Visit	1	14.45	11.32*
Presentation × Visit	1	37.74	29.55*
Patient Gender × Presentation	1	15.39	8.06*
Main Effects			
Physician Gender (M,F)	1	3.99	2.09
Patient Gender (M, F)	1	6.61	3.46
Presentation (somatic, psychosocial)	1	100.75	52.77*
Visit (1,2)	1	24.2	18.94*
Error	130	1.28	

*$p < .05$
[a]Since all terms have one degree of freedom, SS may be omitted (same as MS).
[b]No other interactions reached significance at the $\alpha = .05$ level. All main effects and interactions were included in the reported model. Interpretation of interactions supersedes interpretation of main effects.

minor depression/somatic presentation at both Visit 1 (76% vs. 18%; $\chi^2_{(1)} = 48.3$, $p < .001$) and at Visit 2 (82% vs. 41%; $\chi^2_{(1)} = 24.9$, $p < .001$). Over the two visits, no statistically significant physician or patient gender differences in prescribing behavior were detected with the major depression/psychosocial case. However, with the minor depression/somatic case, male physicians prescribed antidepressants for 26% of male patients and for 62% of female patients ($\chi^2_{(1)} = 6.1$, $p = .01$), while female physicians prescribed antidepressants nearly equivalently to both male and female patients (36% vs. 46%; $\chi^2_{(1)} < 1$, n.s.).

Counseling was suggested more often for the major depression/psychosocial case than for the minor depression/somatic case at both Visit 1 (35% vs. 16%; $\chi^2_{(1)} = 7.1$, $p < .01$) and at Visit 2 (40% vs. 22%; $\chi^2_{(1)} = 5.5$, $p < .01$). Over the two visits, male physicians suggested counseling far more often when the patient was female, with the major depression/psychosocial presentation almost twice as often (59% vs. 30%; $\chi^2_{(1)} = 3.8$, $p < .05$) and with the minor depression/somatic presentation greater than ten times as often (4% vs. 42%; $\chi^2_{(1)} = 10.9$, $p < .001$). Significant differences were not detected in the frequency with which female physicians prescribed antidepressant therapy or suggested counseling to male and female patients, but with the minor depression/somatic case, female physicians recommended counseling significantly more often to female patients (62% vs. 18%; $\chi^2_{(1)}$ = 4.6, p < .03).

As hypothesized, the major depression/psychosocial case and female patients received more prescriptions and recommendations for counseling. However, contrary to expectation, treatment recommendation for male patients varied by physician gender, with male physicians infrequently prescribing medications and both male and female physicians rarely suggesting counseling to male patients.

Notation of Depression in the Medical Chart

By the end of two medical visits, female physicians had noted depression in the charts of nearly all patients, male and female, who presented with major depression and a psychosocial complaint and in the charts of nearly three-quarters of all patients, male and female, who presented with minor depression and a somatic complaint. Likewise, by the close of the second visit, male physicians noted depression in greater than 90% of the charts of both male and female major depression/psychosocial presentation patients. However, they noted depression in charts of fewer than 45% of male and greater than 90% of female somatic presentation patients ($\chi^2_{(1)}$ = 13.6, p < .001). This finding was unexpected in light of the absence of a significant difference in the thoroughness of their exploration of depression with male and female patients (as noted above), although it is consistent with their greater frequency of antidepressant prescriptions and suggestions for counseling for female patients. It is noteworthy that fewer than one in five physicians' chart notations made a distinction between minor and major depression in either patient case.

CONCLUSION

This study of the recognition and treatment of depression in primary care is strengthened by several design features: the use of standardized patients, not one but two medical encounters, two types of depression presentation, and a design which permitted investigation of the influence of physician and patient gender combinations. The findings may be limited, however, by our sampling method which made no attempt to choose a sample representative of primary care physicians in general or at any one of the research sites. While the unpaid volunteer sample was comprised of physicians interested in engaging in primary care research, it is important to note that they were unaware of the project's mental health focus. A further limitation is that although SP intra-performance reliabilities were monitored at each site, no formal agreement statistics were calculated.

Several findings in this study stand out. First, in our study physicians' inquiries about depression symptoms and psychosocial issues and their discussions with patients about the etiology and prognosis of depression were more frequent than earlier reports would suggest (Katon et al., 1986; Katon, Kleinman & Rosen, 1982), though our rates are consistent with those in a recent report by Simon and Von Korff (Simon et al., 1995). Half of the physicians in this study were visited by a patient who presented with two criterion symptoms of depression, inability to concentrate and insomnia, in addition to many associated stressors. As expected, nearly all physicians presented with this case spent more time with the patient and more thoroughly explored depression than their colleagues presented with the minor depression/somatic presentation case, but they also initiated treatment during the first visit. Contrary to expectation, however, well over half of the physicians visited by the milder yet more difficult diagnostic case, the "masked" somatic presentation, both detected and treated the patient's depression. While these latter rates appear consistent with the literature on major depression, they were higher than anticipated for detection and treatment of minor depression (Schulberg et al., 1985; Simon et al., 1995).

It is possible that physicians who agreed to participate in this research are not representative of primary care physicians in general. While we can only speculate about that, there are research design issues and social forces external to earlier studies which offer a context in which to interpret these findings. In prior studies "recognition" of depression was typically operationalized as a notation of depression in the medical chart (Moore, Silimperi & Bobula, 1978; Neilsen & Williams, 1980; Rand, Badger & Coggins, 1988; Zung, Magill, Moore & George, 1983). However, it has been established that mental health diagnoses in medical records imperfectly reflect recognition for a variety of reasons, including associated stigma, difficulty with reimbursement, and the confounding of recognition and record-keeping practices (Burnum, 1989; Robbins et al., 1994). In their favor, chart-based studies can be conducted without priming physicians to "think psychiatrically," in contrast to studies of "recognition" that involve comparison of a physician's assessments of the presence or absence of depression with either a depression screen or with a psychiatrist's evaluation (Gerber et al., 1989; Linzer et al., 1996; Shapiro et al., 1987). This study attempted to resolve these methodological problems. We controlled the validity of a depressive disorder by scripting our standardized patients. We also substantially broadened the definition of "recognition" to take into account the many avenues and domains that may be explored during the medical encounter before diagnostic decisions and chart notations are made. This broader and more satisfactory definition may partially explain the increase of recognition found here.

Over the past decade there have been determined efforts by the National Institute of Mental Health (D/ART Program), as well as by the press, to heighten awareness of the severity of untreated depression. Meanwhile, new pharmacological options such as the Selective Serotonin Reuptake Inhibiters (SSRIs) have been developed and widely publicized. These medications provide physicians with treatments that are both effective and less burdened than their predecessors by troublesome side-effects. Together with the publication of the *Guidelines for the Treatment of Depression in Primary Care* (Panel, 1993), these events may have created a climate in which a diagnosis of depression is more readily made by physicians and accepted by patients.

Other noteworthy findings in this study are the clinical implications suggested by the statistically significant physician-patient gender interactions. Our standardized patients were both standardized and randomly assigned to physicians, thus avoiding any bias attributable to variability in health status and "real" patients' reported desires to be seen by a physician of a given gender. Male and female patients' behaviors, symptoms, and psychosocial histories were pre-scripted to be the same and all met symptom criteria. Despite this, and contrary to our hypotheses, analysis revealed distinct differences between male and female physicians in their handling of female patients. Before interpreting those gender differences, however, it should be noted that the hypothesized greater duration of time female physicians spent with patients was not significantly related to more thorough exploration of depression and psychosocial stressors. When they encounter DSM depression symptoms, exemplified by our major depression/psychosocial presentation, male and female physicians were similar in their approaches to both male and female patients regarding exploration, discussion, and medication. However, there were clear contrasts with regard to referral for on-going counseling. Male physicians suggested counseling more often for female than male patients, whereas female physicians appeared to treat male and female patients in the same way.

While all indices of recognition were less frequent and less thorough with the minor depression/somatic presentation, additional gender patterns occurred. Male physicians visited by male patients discussed depression with 44% of them, prescribed antidepressants for 26% of them, and recommended counseling to 4% of them, whereas, when visited by female patients, male physicians discussed depression with 92% of them, prescribed antidepressants for 62% of them, and recommended counseling for 46% of them. Among female physicians, only recommendations for counseling differed significantly between male and female patients. In fact, female doctors recommended counseling to female patients over three times more frequently than to male patients. Numerous studies have shown that the prevalence of depression among women is twice the prevalence among men, and since this patient's young age was consistent with a high likelihood of a first depressive episode, vigilance was warranted. Physicians in our study were clearly ready to consider and treat depression in their female patients, and yet options for treatment were shaped by both the physicians' and patients' genders.

In this study a diagnosis of depression was often based upon fewer than four DSM criterion symptoms and there was no chart evidence that physicians made a distinction between major and minor depression. As expected, recognition was more frequent for the more severe depression case with the psychosocial presentation (perhaps evidence of the validity of physicians' clinical competence in observing functional status) than for the minor depression case with a somatic presentation. Yet, this study revealed an unanticipated readiness to prescribe antidepressants to patients, especially women, with even mild depression. While awaiting the results of clinical trials of the efficacy of antidepressants for these patients with minor depression, alternative treatment such as counseling, or even no treatment at all, might be as appropriate (Roberts, 1994). The infrequent recommendation of counseling for male patients also warrants further investigation to determine whether physicians anticipate a negative reaction from them (e.g., refusal to attend) or doubt the clinical benefit of counseling for men altogether. Medical research should identify and medical education should address any unconscious social or gender influences that affect the quality and equivalence of medical care (Safran et al., 1997).

REFERENCES

Ashworth, C. D., Williamson, P., & Montano, D. (1984). A scale to measure physician beliefs about psychosocial aspects of patient care. *Soc Sci Med, 19*, 1235-1238.

Badger, L. W., DeGruy, F. V., Hartman, J., Plant, M. A., Leeper, J., Anderson, R., Ficken, R., Gaskins, S., Maxwell, A., Rand, E., & Tietze, P. (1994). Patient Presentation, Interview Content, and the Detection of Depression by Primary Care Physicians. *Psychosomatic Medicine, 56*, 128-135.

Barrett, J. E., Barrett, J. A., Oxman, T. E., & Gerber, P. D. (1988). The prevalence of psychiatric disorders in a primary care practice. *Arch Gen Psychiatry, 45*, 1100-1106.

Baughman, O. (1994). Rapid diagnosis and treatment of anxiety and depression in primary care: The somatizing patient. *Journal of Family Practice, 39*(4), 373-378.

Bernzweig, J., Takayama, J. I., Phibbs, C., Lewis, C., & Pantell, R. H. (1997). Gender differences in physician-patient communication. Evidence from pediatric visits. *Archives of Pediatric Adolescent Medicine, 151*(6), 586-91.

Bertakis, K. D., Helms, L. J., Callahan, E. J., Azari, R., & Robbins, J. A. (1995). The influence of gender on physician practice style. *Medical Care, 33*(4), 406-416.

Burns, B. J., & Burke, J. D. (1985). Improving mental health practices in primary care: Findings from recent research. *Public Health Reports, 100,* 294-300.

Burnum, J. F. (1989). The misinformation era: The fall of the medical record. *Annals of Internal Medicine, 110,* 482-484.

Campbell, J. D., Neikirk, H. K., & Hosokawa, M. C. (1990). Development of a psychosocial concern index from videotaped interviews of nurse practitioners and family physicians. *Journal of Family Practice, 30,* 321-326.

Eisenberg, L. (1992). Treating depression and anxiety in primary care. *N Eng J Med, 326*(16), 1080-1084.

Froom, J. (1988). Mental disorders in primary care. *Lancet, Dec,* 1371.

Gerber, P. D., Barrett, J. E., Barrett, J. A., Manheimer, E., Whiting, R., & Smith, R. (1989). Recognition of depression by internists in primary care: A comparison of internist and "gold standard" psychiatric assessments. *Journal of General Internal Medicine, 4,* 7-13.

Goldberg, D., Steele, J. J., Johnson, A., & Smith, C. (1982). Ability of primary care physicians to make accurate rating of psychiatric symptoms. *Ann Gen Psychiatry, 39,* 829-833.

Hall, J. A., Irish, J. T., Roter, D. L. et al. (1994a). Gender in medical encounters: An analysis of physician and patient communication in a primary care setting. *Health Psychology, 13,* 384-392.

Hall, J. A., Irish, J. T., Roter, D. L. et al. (1994b). Satisfaction, gender, and communication in medical visits. *Medical Care, 32,* 1216-1231.

Hoeper, E. W., Nycz, G. R., Cleary, P. O. et al. (1979). Estimated prevalence of RDC mental disorder in primary care. *International Journal of Mental Health, 8,* 6-15.

Katon, W., Berg, A. O., Robins, A. J. et al. (1986). Depression: Medical utilization and somatization. *Western Journal of Medicine, 144,* 564-568.

Katon, W., Kleinman, A., & Rosen, G. (1982). Depression and somatization: A review. Part I. *Am J Med, 72,* 127-135.

Katon, W., Kleinman, A., & Rosen, G. (1982). Depression and somatization: A review. Part II. *Am J Med, 72,* 241-247.

Katon, W., & Schulberg, H. (1992). Epidemiology of depression in primary care. *Gen Hosp Psychiatry, 14,* 237-247.

Kerssens, J. J., Bensing, J. M., & Andela, M. G. (1997). Patient preference for genders of health professionals. *Social Science in Medicine, 44,* 1531-1540.

Kirk, R.E. (1995) Experimental Design: Procedures for the Behavioral Sciences (3rd Edition). Pacific Grove, CA: Brooks/Cole Publishing Company.

Kirmayer, L. J., Robbins, J. M., Dworkin, M., & Yaffe, M. J. (1993). Somatization and the recognition of depression and anxiety in primary care. *American Journal of Psychiatry, 150*(5), 734-741.

Linzer, M., Spitzer, R., Williams, J. B. W., Hahn, S., Brody, D., & deGruy, F. (1996). Gender: Quality of life, and mental disorders in primary care: Results from the PRIME-MD 1000 study. *American Journal of Medicine, 101,* 526-533.

Mathew, R. J., Weinman, M. L., & Mirabi, M. (1981). Physical symptoms of depression. *Brit J Psychiatry, 139,* 293-296.

Moore, J. T., Silimperi, D. R., & Bobula, J. A. (1978). Recognition of depression by family practice residents: The impact of screening. *Journal of Family Practice, 7*, 509-513.

Neilsen, A. C., & Williams, T. A. (1980). Depression in ambulatory care: Prevalence by self-report questionnaire and recognition by non-psychiatric physicians. *Archives of General Psychiatry, 37*, 999-1004.

Novack, D. H., Goldberg, R. J., Rowland-Morin, P., Landau, C., & Wartman, S. (1989). Toward a comprehensive psychiatry/behavioral science curriculum for primary care residents. *Psychosomatics, 30*, 213-223.

Panel, D. G. (1993). *Depression in Primary Care: Volume 1. Detection and Diagnosis Clinical Practice Guideline, Number 5.* Rockville, MD. U.S. Department of Health and Human Services, Public Health Service, Agency for Health Care Policy and Research. Paper presented at the AHCPR Publication.

Pardes, H. (1979). The provision of mental health services in primary care settings. In *Mental Health Services in General Health Care, Volume 1.*

Rand, E. H., Badger, L. W., & Coggins, D. (1988). Toward a resolution of contradictions: Utility of feedback from the GHQ. *General Hospital Psychiatry, 10*, 189-196.

Robbins, J. M., Kirmayer, L. J., Cathebras, P., Yaffe, M. J., & Dworkind, M. (1994). Physician characteristics and the recognition of depression and anxiety in primary care. *Medical Care, 32*(8), 795-812.

Roberts, S. J. (1994). Somatization in primary care. The common presentation of psychosocial problems through physical complaints. *Nurse Practitioner, 19*(5), 47, 50-56.

Roter, D., Lipkin, M., & Korsgard, A. (1991). Sex differences in patients' and physicians' communication during primary care medical visits. *Medical Care, 29*, 1083-1093.

Safran, D. G., Rogers, W. H., Tarlov, A. R., McHorney, C. A., & Ware, J. E., Jr. (1997). Gender differences in medical treatment: The case of physician-prescribed activity restrictions. *Social Science in Medicine, 45*(5), 711-722.

Schulberg, H. C., McClelland, M., & Coulehan, J. L. (1986). Psychiatric decision-making in family practice: Future research directions. *General Hospital Psychiatry, 8*, 1-6.

Schulberg, H. C., & McClelland, M. A. (1987). A conceptual model for educating primary care providers in the diagnosis and treatment of depression. *General Hospital Psychiatry, 9*, 1-10.

Schulberg, H. C., Saul, M., McClelland, M., Ganguli, M., Christy, W., & Frank, R. (1985). Assessing depression in primary medical and psychiatric practices. *Arch Gen Psychiatry, 42*, 1164-1170.

Shapiro, S., German, P. S., Skinnner, E. A., VonKorff, M., Turner, R. W., Klein, L. E., Teitelbaum, M. L., Kramer, M., Burke, J., & Burns, B. J. (1987). An experiment to change detection and management of mental morbidity in primary care. *Medical Care, 25*, 327-339.

Simon, G. E., Ormel, J., VonKorff, M., & Barlow, W. (1995). Health care costs associated with depressive and anxiety disorders in primary care. *American Journal of Psychiatry, 152*, 352-357.

Verbrugge, L. M. (1984). How physicians treat mentally distressed men and women. *Social Science in Medicine, 18*(1), 1-9.

Wallen, J., Waitzkin, H., & Stoeckle, J. D. (1979). Physicians' stereotypes about female health and illness: A study of patient's sex and the information process during medical interviews. *Women's Health, 4*, 135.

Weisman, C., & Teitelbaum, M. A. (1985). Physician gender and the physician-patient relationship: Recent evidence and relevant questions. *Social Science and Medicine, 20*(11), 1119-1127.

Williams, J. B. W., Spitzer, R., Linzer, M., Kroenke, K., Hahn, S., DeGruy, F. V., & Lazev, A. (1995). Gender differences in depression in primary care. *American Journal of Obstetrics and Gynecology, 173*, 654-9.

Zung, W. W. K., Magill, M., Moore, J. T., & George, D. T. (1983). Recognition and treatment of depression in a family medicine practice. *Journal of Clinical Psychiatry, 44*, 3-6.

Reactivity and Responsiveness in Children's Service Systems

William R. Nugent
Charles Glisson

SUMMARY. Few studies have examined the extent to which public children's service systems respond to the mental health problems of children in state custody. This is an important issue because previous research suggests that little attention is given to children's mental health service needs when judicial and service decisions are made about children who enter state custody. The current study addresses the issue by examining the extent to which one state's children's service system is responsive versus reactive to the mental health problems of the children in its care. A responsive system is one in which services are provided to meet each child's unique mental health needs. A reactive system is one in which service providers take actions to avoid providing needed mental health services. Our results describe a service system that is more reactive than responsive to children's mental health problems. *[Article copies available for a fee from The Haworth Document Delivery Service: 1-800-342-9678. E-mail address: getinfo@haworthpressinc.com]*

KEYWORDS. Children's service systems, mental health services, system responsiveness, system reactivity

William R. Nugent is Associate Professor, Children's Mental Health Services Research Center, The University of Tennessee, Knoxville. Charles Glisson is Professor and Director, Children's Mental Health Services Research Center, The University of Tennessee, Knoxville.

This research was supported by NIMH grants MH 46124 and MH 53623.

[Haworth co-indexing entry note]: "Reactivity and Responsiveness in Children's Service Systems." Nugent, William R., and Charles Glisson. Co-published simultaneously in *Journal of Social Service Research* (The Haworth Press, Inc.) Vol. 25, No. 3, 1999, pp. 41-60; and: *Mental Health Services and Sectors of Care* (ed: Enola K. Proctor, Nancy Morrow-Howell, and Arlene Stiffman) The Haworth Press, Inc., 1999, pp. 41-60. Single or multiple copies of this article are available for a fee from The Haworth Document Delivery Service [1-800-342-9678, 9:00 a.m. - 5:00 p.m. (EST). E-mail address: getinfo@haworthpressinc.com].

41

Almost one million children are estimated to be in the custody of the nation's child welfare and juvenile justice systems (Barth et al., 1994; Center for the Study of Social Policy, 1990, 1993; National Center on Child Abuse and Neglect, 1996). In Tennessee the number of children in state custody has doubled over the past decade, with approximately 12,000 children currently in the custody of the State of Tennessee. Throughout the nation, it has become increasingly evident that public child welfare and juvenile justice systems serving children in custody are in crisis. The documented levels of neglect, emotional disorder and antisocial behavior that characterize many of these children's lives create serious risks for the children, their families, and their communities. These risks emphasize the need for effective and efficient service systems that are responsive to the individual needs of each child (Schorr, 1997; Stroul & Friedman, 1996).

Children entering state custody are especially at risk of chronic, long term mental health problems that can follow them into adulthood. Although these risks are of most concern to both the child's welfare and the community, the risks are not given adequate consideration in the services the children receive (Henggeler, 1994; Lindsey, 1994; National Advisory Mental Health Council, 1990; Rosenblatt & Attkinson, 1992). Regardless of the reason for custody, many children enter state custody with a variety of mental health-related problems, including multiple diagnoses (Behar, 1985; Dougherty et al., 1987; Duchnowski & Friedman, 1990; Frank, 1980; Kashani et al., 1987; Rosenfeld et al., 1997). In fact, some of the most serious mental health problems that affect children can be found among those who enter state custody (Glisson, 1996; Kahn & Kamerman, 1992; Knitzer & Yelton, 1990; Rosenfeld et al., 1997). All of this points to the importance of ensuring that children in state custody receive services that address their individual mental health needs. In spite of these problems and concerns, few studies have investigated how public children's service systems respond to children's mental health problems (Thompson & Wilcox, 1995). While research on the role that mental health plays in service decisions and service provision for children in state custody has been identified as a national research priority for some time, to date little research has been conducted (National Advisory Mental Health Council, 1990).

In one of the few studies completed to date, Glisson (1996) showed that the mental health service needs of children are unrelated to either the judicial or service decisions made on their behalf as they enter custody. The key characteristics related to judicial and service decisions were the child's age, gender, and, to a lesser extent, the number of times the child had previously been in custody. The children's mental health problems were unrelated to mental health service decisions, although Glisson (1996) found that the majority of the children entering custody had clinically significant mental health problems. However, only 14% actually received mental health services and there was no relationship between the children's need and receipt of services. In addition, proportionately fewer minority children received mental health services (8%), although the level of need was similar to that of non-minority children.

While this and other research has demonstrated the limited role that mental health plays in decisions made on behalf of children as they enter custody, more research is needed to fully understand how service systems respond to children's mental health problems. Ideally, a service system should be responsive to the mental health profile of each child it serves (Behar, 1985; Henggeler, 1994; Stroul & Friedman, 1996). The most common child and adolescent mental health problem profiles brought to the attention of professionals are those that involve antisocial (or so-called "externalizing") behavior, such as aggression, stealing, and disobedience (Kazdin, 1995; McMahon, 1994; Weisz et al., 1997). The second most common type of mental health problem profiles involve "internalizing" emotional and behavioral problems, such as depression, anxiety, and relationship difficulties with other children (Ollendick & King, 1994; Weisz et al., 1997). Often these two types of problems are comorbid in children and adolescents (Alessi & Magen, 1988; Anderson et al., 1987; Elliott et al., 1989). The interventions used for these different problems in children and adolescents seem to produce important specific effects, with effect sizes for specific target problems about twice as large as they are for related but non-specific target problems (Weisz et al., 1997). Further, there is evidence that children and adolescents who are manifesting concurrent internalizing and externalizing problems may be at particularly high risk for negative outcomes (McMahon, 1994) and may show differential reactions to intervention procedures (Ollendick & King, 1994). These characteristics of the mental health problems experienced by children and adolescents, as well as of the intervention procedures used to treat these problems, makes it critical that a service system respond specifically and appropriately to a child's externalizing and internalizing problem levels.

RESPONSIVENESS IN SERVICE SYSTEMS

The above underscores the importance of the responsiveness of a children's service system. The *Webster's Ninth New Collegiate Dictionary* (1990) defines the word "responsive" as a quickness to respond appropriately or sympathetically. In a responsive system, services are provided quickly and appropriately to each child in a manner that is sensitive to the child's profile of internalizing and externalizing mental health problems. That is, children with more serious internalizing problems should be more likely to receive mental health and related support services, and children with more serious externalizing problems should be more likely to receive mental health and related support services. Further, the magnitude of these relationships should be equal. These equal relationships represent the service system's sensitive, sympathetic response to children's unique needs, with equal importance given to internalizing and externalizing mental health problems.

REACTIVITY IN SERVICE SYSTEMS

In previous research, findings suggested that service sectors in Tennessee's children's service system competed with one another to avoid providing services to the most problematic children (Glisson, 1994; Glisson & James, 1992). Children with more severe mental health problems, particularly externalizing problems, were found to experience numerous residential placements and placement ejections. These problems resulted in service providers attempting to avoid accepting responsibility for these more problematic children, with case manager requests for services for these children being more and more frequently refused. As a result of these refusals, case managers had to seek services for these children farther and farther from their home communities.

These observations and other previous research led us to develop the concept of "system reactivity." "React" is defined as acting in opposition to a force or condition and "reaction" is a contrary or opposing action, as an action induced by vital resistance to something else, such as the response of tissue to a foreign substance (*Webster's II New Riverside University Dictionary*, 1984; *Webster's Ninth New Collegiate Dictionary*, 1990). Our concept of "system reactivity" refers to patterns in service systems in which the systems act in opposition to children's behavioral and mental health problems, reducing the likelihood that the children will receive the services they need. The more reactive systems reject or eject children who present the most challenge and require the most attention and resources. It is as if these systems deem a particular input (i.e., a child with a certain psychosocial profile) as undesirable and try to pass the input through the system "unprocessed." In this context, unprocessed means "without providing needed services." Indicators of system reactivity might be any of the following responses to children's mental health needs: refusals by service providers to provide needed services, interrupting and stopping the provision of certain services before they have been completed, and repeated residential placements that are disrupted prior to service completion. Service system reactivity may be iatrogenic since repeated placement and service disruptions may place a child at even greater risk of serious mental health problems (Behar, 1985; Curry et al., 1988).

THE RELATIONSHIP BETWEEN RESPONSIVENESS AND REACTIVITY

The notions of responsiveness and reactivity allow us to elaborate on earlier observations that elements of children's service systems compete to avoid providing services to the most problematic children in state custody. This effort to avoid providing services to certain children implies a reciprocal and negative relationship between responsiveness and reactivity. The more a service system reacts to a child–by numerous service disruptions, placement ejections, service refusals, etc.–the less likely it is to be responsive to the child's needs. In turn, the lack of service provision exacerbates system reactivity, in part because the child's mental health needs are ignored, which is likely to increase the child's psychosocial problems and make the child even less acceptable to the service system (Kazdin, 1995; McMahon, 1994; Ollendick & King, 1994). In contrast, when a system provides appropriate services in response to a child's mental health needs, the child's psychosocial problems can be stabilized or reduced and the reactivity of the system decreases. And, in a continuing cycle, the more the reactivity decreases, the more the responsiveness of the system increases.

RESEARCH HYPOTHESES

The current study focuses on the relationships between children's demographic characteristics (age and gender), the children's mental health problems (internalizing and externalizing behavior) upon entry into state custody, and the reactivity and responsiveness of the public children's service system. Several hypotheses were tested in this research and these hypotheses are embodied in the structural model shown in Figure 1. The specific hypotheses tested are as follows:

1. The children's service system will be reactive to both internalizing and externalizing problems, but more reactive to externalizing problems.
2. The children's service system is unresponsive to children's internalizing and externalizing problems.
3. There is a reciprocal relationship between system responsiveness and system reactivity.
4. Age and gender are related to children's internalizing and externalizing problems at entry into custody, with older children and males presenting more serious problems.
5. Age and gender are related to system reactivity such that the system is more reactive to males and older children.

FIGURE 1. Hypothesized structural model for the children's service system in Tennessee. The + and − signs indicate path coefficients with predicted positive or negative signs, respectively. The paths marked with ns indicate those predicted to be statistically nonsignificant.

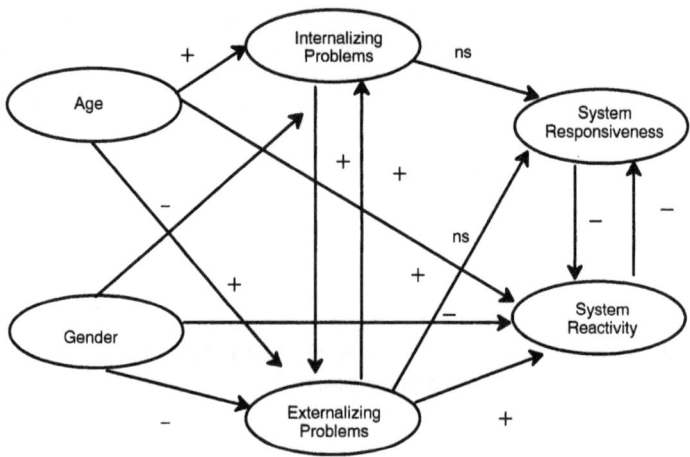

In the model shown in Figure 1 we have modeled a reciprocal relationship between children's internalizing and externalizing problems at entry into custody. We chose to model this relationship on the basis of evidence that internalizing and externalizing problems frequently coexist in children and adolescents (Bernstein & Borchardt, 1991; Harrington et al., 1991; King et al., 1990; Kovacs et al., 1988; Ryan et al., 1987). However, there were other ways in which the relationship between internalizing and externalizing problems could be modeled and these different representations were included in several alternate models we tested. As will be seen below, the results of tests of the above hypotheses did not depend on the manner in which the relationship between internalizing and externalizing problems was modeled.

In hypothesis (2) we speculated that the children's service system is nonresponsive to children's mental health problems. In the model shown in Figure 1, however, we included direct paths from internalizing problems and externalizing problems to system responsiveness in order to directly test the extent to which the children's service system is responsive. Consistent with earlier discussion, we constrained these paths to be equal in magnitude. Our hypothesis implied that these two paths should be statistically nonsignificant.

Some previous research suggests that children's service systems may function differently in providing mental health services for minority children than for non-minority children (Glisson, 1994, 1996). This possibility was tested in the current research by testing the invariance of the hypothesized model over subsamples of non-minority and minority children (Bryne, 1995; Joreskog & Sorbom, 1993).

METHODOLOGY

The study sampled children served by the Tennessee Departments of Human Services (DHS) and of Youth Development (DYD) in 28 rural and urban counties. It should be noted that subsequent to this research, the two departments' children's service systems were merged to form a single children's service department. The systematic sample of 718 children and adolescents was obtained from those placed in the custody of the state of Tennessee for abuse, neglect, status offenses, or delinquency. We tracked prospectively the services and placements provided to children for one year following their date of entry into custody. Approximately 85% remained in custody longer than three months, 75% longer than six months and 51% were still in custody after one year. Only children over the age of four were included in the sample because of the difficulty in assessing the psychosocial functioning of preschool children.

A measurement model was developed in which both single indicator and multiple indicators were used to represent constructs. Single indicators were used to represent the constructs of age and gender (Williams, 1996), while multiple indicators were used to represent the constructs of internalizing problems, externalizing problems, system reactivity, and system responsiveness. While no empirical methods were used to estimate the reliabilities of recordings of subjects' age and gender, it seemed reasonable to assume that both variables were recorded with a small amount of error. Thus, the reliabilities of both of these measures were arbitrarily estimated to be about .95 (Hayduk, 1987; Williams, 1996).

As children entered state custody their psychosocial functioning was assessed using both the Child Behavior Checklist (CBCL) completed by parents or parent surrogates, and the Teacher's Report Form (TRF) completed by their teachers (Achenbach, 1991a, b). Scores from the Externalizing and Internalizing scales of the CBCL and TRF were used in the analyses described below. The coefficient alpha estimates of reliability for these scales were .91 for the Internalizing scales of both CBCL and TRF; .94 for CBCL Externalizing scores; and .96 for TRF Externalizing scores. Achenbach (1991a, b) presents evidence for the validity of both Internalizing and Externalizing scales of the CBCL and TRF with both clinical and nonclinical populations.

Internalizing problems were measured as the subjects' CBCL and TRF Internalizing Scale T-scores, while externalizing problems were measured as the subject's CBCL and TRF Externalizing Scale T-scores. Using both the CBCL and TRF provides indicators of more generalized internalizing and externalizing problems than would either the CBCL or TRF scores alone. Achenbach (1991a, b) and others have noted that reports of children's behavior problems by parents and teachers correlate poorly and that children's behavior problems in school and home settings may be context bound. Measuring internalizing and externalizing problems as the commonality between parent and teacher reports creates a construct representing problems that are consistent across situations, as opposed to problems that are specific to particular settings.

A number of measures of the functioning of the children's service system were used in the present study: number of mental health services received, number of nonmental health services received, number of placements for the child or adolescent, number of placement ejections experienced by the child, number of times that service providers refused to provide requested services for the child or adolescent, and proximity of the child's placement to the child's home community. These measures were obtained from the records of case managers who were responsible for the children in the study sample. Reliability analyses of our record review procedures have suggested interrater reliabilities between .78 and .96 (Nugent et al., 1998).

Indicators of System Responsiveness

"Number of mental health services received" and "number of nonmental health services received" were used as indicators of system responsiveness in the analyses described below. "Number of mental health services received" was defined as the numerical sum of the following services received by the child over the period the child was tracked: individual counseling or psychotherapy, group counseling or psychotherapy, family counseling or therapy, drug abuse treatment, and alcohol abuse treatment. "Number of nonmental health services received" was defined as the numerical sum of services such as educational services, transportation services, medical services, etc., received by the child while in custody.

Indicators of System Reactivity

Four variables were used as indicators of system reactivity in the measurement model. "Number of placement ejections" experienced by the child was defined as the total number of times the child was removed from a service placement due to reasons of inappropriate behavior or untreatable characteristics. "Number of placements" was defined as the total number of service placements the child entered during the course of the twelve months the child was tracked. "Number of service refusals" was defined as the total number of times that service providers refused to provide requested services for the child. "Proximity of services" was defined as the distance in miles between the child's last placement and the child's home community.

The measurement model was fitted to non-minority and minority subsamples separately using the multiple groups method (Joreskog & Sorbom, 1993a; Byrne, 1995). It was necessary to fix some parameters associated with constructs represented by only one or two indicators in order to facilitate estimation (Hoyle & Panter, 1995). The loading of number of mental health services received on system responsiveness was set at 1.0 as was the loading of number of placement ejections on system reactivity (Joreskog & Sorbom, 1993a). The loading of TRF Internalizing Scale T-scores on internalizing problems was set at 1.0, and the loading of TRF Externalizing Scale T-scores on externalizing problems was set at 1.0 (Hoyle & Panter, 1995; Joreskog & Sorbom, 1993a).

Ordinal Variables

The indicators, "number of mental health services received" and "number of nonmental health services received," were numerical counts of the number of different services received by each child. However, neither of these variables indicated the full extent of the services received by children because information about the specific services was not included in these counts. For example, the specific number of individual counseling sessions a child attended was not included in the numerical count that comprises "number of mental health services received." Hence, the variables "number of mental health services received" and "number of nonmental health services received" were treated as ordinal variables using the program PRELIS 2 (Joreskog & Sorbom, 1992b).

The variables "number of placement ejections," "number of placements," and "number of service refusals" were all skewed, kurtotic, and showed evidence of floor effects as can be seen in Table 1. Thus, these variables were treated as being censored below (Joreskog & Sorbom, 1993b). The program PRELIS 2 (Joreskog & Sorbom, 1993b) was used to transform these variables in order to reduce their nonnormality. Following suggestions of Joreskog and Sorbom (1993a, b), a matrix of Pearson, polyserial, and tetrachoric correlations was computed and used as input into LISREL 8 and weighted least squares methods used in all analyses. Weighted least squares was used because of the substantial evidence of violations of the distribution-

TABLE 1. Sample Characteristics

Non-Minority Children	mean	SD	SK	K
Age	14.45	2.6	−1.25	1.48
CBCL Internalizing T-score	62.5	12.4	−0.35	−0.27
CBCL Externalizing T-score	67.7	13.4	−0.47	−0.27
TRF Internalizing T-score	60.4	10.4	−0.18	0.76
TRF Externalizing T-score	63.4	10.9	0.04	−0.18
Placements	4.3	2.9	1.1	1
Placement ejections	0.33	0.8	3.4	13.3
Service refusals	1	3.3	6.6	55.6
Mental health services	2.4	1.8	0.72	−0.07
Nonmental health services	2.4	1.8	0.72	−0.07
Distance from home (in miles) of services received	30.4	61	3.1	12.4
Minority Children	mean	SD	SK	K
Age	14.56	3	−1.3	1.96
CBCL Internalizing T-score	61.6	12.5	−0.43	−3.1
CBCL Externalizing T-score	68.3	13	−0.5	−0.1
TRF Internalizing T-score	60.3	10.7	−0.15	1.13
TRF Externalizing T-score	63.7	10.3	0.02	−0.15
Placements	4.8	2.9	1.1	1.1
Placement ejections	0.56	1.3	5	33.1
Service refusals	2	5.5	5.5	37
Mental health services	2.2	1.6	0.39	−1.0
Nonmental health services	2.5	1.7	0.7	0.03
Distance from home (in miles) of services received	46.8	73.6	2.1	4.9

SD = standard deviation; SK = skewness; K = kurtosis

al assumptions of normality seen in the sample characterizations in Table 1 (Joreskog & Sorbom, 1993a).

Data Analysis

We split the sample into two parts: non-minority children and minority children, given prior evidence of differences in service availability. Multiple groups structural equation modeling (SEM) methods (Joreskog & Sorbom, 1993a) were then used to develop a measurement model for the constructs shown in Figure 1: age, gender, internalizing problems, externalizing problems, system responsiveness, and system reactivity. Then the hypothesized structural model shown in Figure 1 was tested by fitting the model to the multiple groups data using LISREL 8 (Joreskog & Sorbom, 1993a).

RESULTS

Sample Characteristics

There were 582 cases in the subsample of non-minority children. In this subsample, 339 of the children were male (58.3%) and 243 were female (41.7%). There were 136 cases in the subsample of minority children. Eighty-one (81) of these children were male (59.6%), and 55 were female (40.4%). Distributional indices for several variables for both non-minority and minority children in the sample are shown in Table 1.

Sample Comparability

The non-minority and minority subsamples were compared to determine the extent to which they were statistically similar. The results suggest that the subsamples differed significantly on only three variables: number of placement ejections, number of service referrals, and proximity of services. On all three of these variables minority children had significantly higher means.

Tests of Measurement Model

The Chi-square for the test of invariance of the measurement model across the two samples was $\chi^2(121, N = 718) = 233.23$, $p < .00001$; Goodness-of-Fit Index (GFI) = .90, Incremental-Fit Index (IFI) = .96, Comparative-Fit Index (CFI) = .96, Critical N (CN) = 492 (Hoyle & Panter, 1995). Modification indices suggested setting the path from system reactivity to number of service refusals free in the minority sample. This change resulted in a model χ^2 (120, N = 718) = 214.00, $p < .00001$; GFI = .91, IFI = .96, CFI = .96, CN = 533. The model change Chi-square was $\chi^2(1) = 19.23$ ($p < .00001$). Modification indices further suggested setting the path from system reactivity to proximity of services free in the minority sample. This change resulted in a model $\chi^2(119, N = 718) = 207.97$, $p < .00001$; GFI = .91, IFI = .97, CFI = .97, CN = 554. The model change Chi-square was $\chi^2(1) = 6.03$ ($p < .015$). Modification indices also suggested setting the error covariance between CBCL Internalizing and Externalizing scores free in the minority sample. This change resulted in a model $\chi^2(118, N = 718) = 194.72$, p = .000011; GFI = .92, IFI = .97, CFI = .97, CN = 577. The model change Chi-square was $\chi^2(1) = 13.25$ (p < .0003). At this point no further changes in the measurement model were indicated. Several alternate measurement models were tested, but none proved to be as good as or superior to the one described here.

The final measurement model for non-minority children is shown in Figure 2, while the final measurement model for minority children is shown in Figure 3. The above results show that the measurement model was not invariant across non-minority and minority subjects (Byrne, 1995). The overall

FIGURE 2. Measurement model for sample of non-minority children. Upper numbers indicate estimated coefficients; middle figures in parentheses indicate standard errors of coefficients; bottom figures indicate t-ratios. All t-ratios greater than 1.96 are statistically significant beyond the .05 level. CBCL = Child Behavior Checklist; TRF = Teacher Report Form; INT = Internalizing Problems; EXT = Externalizing Problems; Gend = gender; MH = number of mental health services received; NMH = number of nonmental health services received; RESP = system responsiveness; EJECT = number of placement ejections; NUMPLAC = number of placements; PROX = proximity of services; REJECT = number of service refusals; REACT = system reactivity.

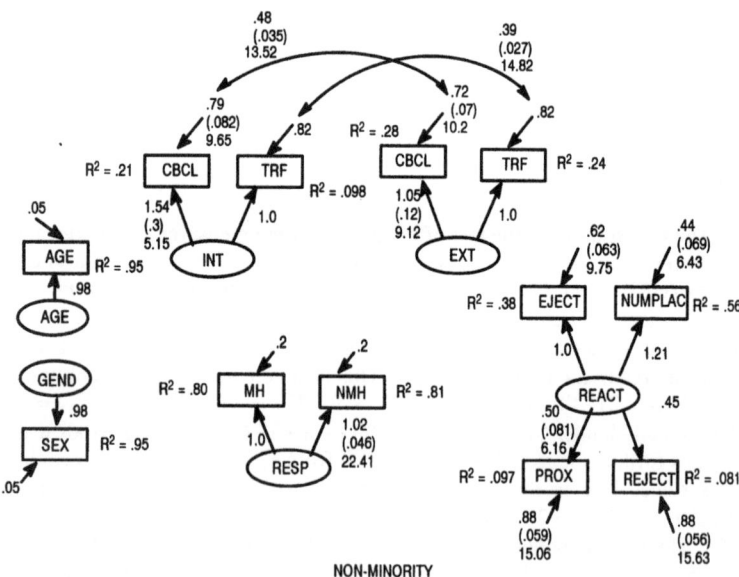

NON-MINORITY

FIGURE 3. Measurement model for sample of minority children. Upper numbers indicate estimated coefficients; middle figures in parentheses indicate standard errors of coefficients; bottom figures indicate t-ratios. All t-ratios greater than 1.96 are statistically significant beyond the .05 level. CBCL = Child Behavior Checklist; TRF = Teacher Report Form; INT = Internalizing Problems; EXT = Externalizing Problems; Gend = gender; MH = number of mental health services received; NMH = number of nonmental health services received; RESP = system responsiveness; EJECT = number of placement ejections; NUMPLAC = number of placements; PROX = proximity of services; REJECT = number of service refusals; REACT = system reactivity.

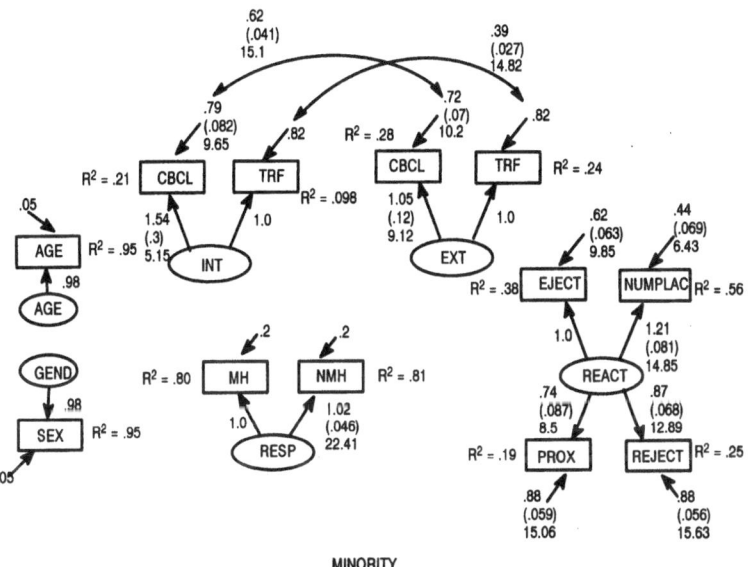

MINORITY

Chi-square change for the three between sample differences was $\chi^2(3) = 38.51$ (p < .00001). The results suggested that, for a given level of system reactivity, minority children were more likely to be refused services and to be placed further from their home community than non-minority children.

Test of Hypothesized Model

The final results of testing the hypothesized structural model are shown in Figure 4. The model chi-square was $\chi^2(136, N = 718) = 197.01$, p = .00049, GFI = .91, CFI = .98, IFI = .98, CN = 645. As can be seen in Figure 4, age had significant direct, positive effects on both internalizing and externalizing

FIGURE 4. Final results of LISREL analysis testing hypothesized structural model. Upper numbers indicate estimated coefficients; middle numbers in parentheses indicate standard errors of estimated coefficients; lower numbers indicate t-ratios. All estimated coefficients that are marked with an asterisk (*) indicate those that are statistically significant.

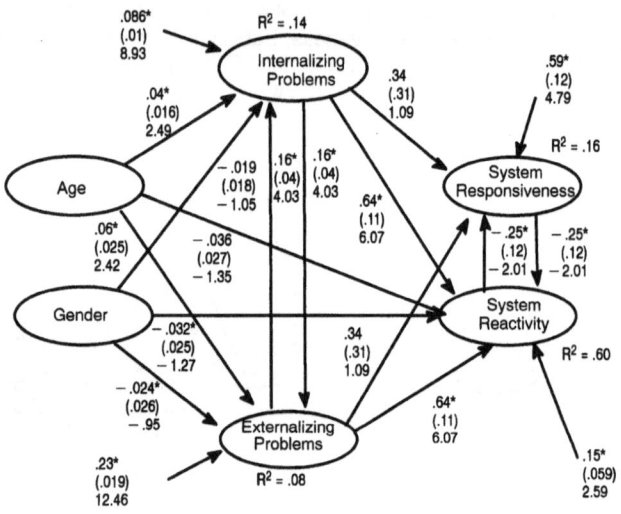

*p < .05

problems, as hypothesized and consistent with Glisson's (1994, 1996) earlier research. However, contrary to expectations, there was no significant direct effect of gender on either internalizing or externalizing problems. There were no significant direct effects of age or gender on system reactivity, contrary to our prediction. As hypothesized, the paths from internalizing problems to responsiveness and from externalizing problems to responsiveness were non-significant. As hypothesized, there was a significant direct positive effect of externalizing problems on system reactivity. There was also a significant direct, positive effect of internalizing problems on system reactivity. The magnitude of the path coefficient from externalizing problems to system reactivity (standardized coefficient = .54) was larger in magnitude than the path from internalizing problems to system reactivity (standardized coefficient = .33). While these results were consistent with our expectations, the difference was statistically nonsignificant [$\chi^2(1)$ = .82, p > .05]. Thus, in the results shown in Figure 4, these paths are constrained to be equal. The results also confirmed the negative reciprocal relationship between system responsiveness and system reactivity discussed earlier. All parameter estimates in this model were within appropriate bounds; there were no out of range values, such as negative (Heywood) error variances, R^2 values greater than 1.0, or standardized covariance estimates greater than 1.0. The stability coefficient for the model was less than one, indicating that the infinite series implied by the reciprocal paths in the model converge (Joreskog & Sorbom, 1993a). Finally, there was no evidence the structural model differed across non-minority and minority samples.

Alternate Structural Models

Several alternate structural models were fitted to the data as a means of testing alternative representatives of the children's service system. Models were tested in which: (1) the paths from internalizing and externalizing problems to system reactivity were unequal; (2) the reciprocal paths between system responsiveness and system reactivity were eliminated; (3) the reciprocal paths between system responsiveness and system reactivity were unequal in magnitude; (4) the paths from internalizing and externalizing problems to system responsiveness were unequal in magnitude; and (5) there were no direct paths from internalizing and externalizing problems to system reactivity. All of these alternate models were significantly worse than the final model described above.

We also tested the sensitivity of the model to changes in the way that internalizing problems and externalizing problems were related to one another. Three alternate possibilities were investigated: (a) one in which internalizing problems directly affected externalizing problems (but not vice versa); (b) one in which externalizing problems directly affected internalizing problems (but not vice versa); and (c) one in which internalizing and externalizing problems were each directly affected by some omitted variable, but neither variable directly affected the other. While the coefficients describing the relationships between these two constructs changed in each alternate model, the other coefficients in the models remained invariant. Thus, the manner in which the relationship between internalizing and externalizing problems was modeled had no effect on the other components of the structural model.

DISCUSSION

The above results are consistent with previous research suggesting that children's mental health problems and service needs do not play a direct role in the children's receipt of services from public children's service systems.

The lack of direct paths from either internalizing problems or externalizing problems to system responsiveness shows the failure of the service system to respond to each child's unique mental health needs. These results expand on earlier research which showed that children's problems in psychosocial functioning were not related to either the judicial decisions upon the child's entry into custody or the initial service decisions made on the child's behalf by service providers.

The direct paths from externalizing and internalizing problems to system reactivity clearly suggest that service providers in the children's service system avoided providing services to children with internalizing mental health problems to the same extent that they avoided providing services to children with externalizing behavior problems. Why this might be true is unclear. Perhaps a child presenting with any apparent mental health problems, whether internalizing or externalizing, poses a problem for the custody system. The manner in which internalizing and externalizing problems were defined in this research–i.e., by the commonality between parent and teacher reports of child problems in psychosocial functioning–created a more generalized conceptualization of psychosocial functioning problems than would definitions using only parent or only teacher reports. Thus, the above results may be descriptive of how the custody system responded and reacted to children whose problems were consistent across situations.

Another possible explanation for the direct path from internalizing problems to system reactivity is a misunderstanding of children's mental health problems by service workers, residential placement staff or foster parents. If behaviors symptomatic of internalizing problems were interpreted as reactions to custody or an inappropriate placement, then the path from internalizing problems to system reactivity could reflect an attempt by service providers to avoid children with mental health problems who were seen to be particularly challenging. A related possibility is that children with internalizing behavior problems exhibit behaviors in placements that are the result of the interaction between their internalizing problems and the demands of the placement setting that again result in efforts of residential staff and others to avoid responsibility for their care. In either case, the adequate training of service workers in the assessment and differential diagnosis of internalizing and externalizing behavior problems, along with training in appropriate treatment protocols, may help decrease system reactivity to children's internalizing problems.

The results indicate that the best way for a child in state custody to receive the most services is for that child not to have any problems in psychosocial functioning. However, as documented earlier, a large proportion of children entering state custody have serious mental health problems. The results shown in Figure 4 also suggest that improving the provision of services to children in custody requires lowering system reactivity to children's mental health problems. This implies, among other things, doing what is necessary to provide stable placements to children who have the most serious problems. The model in Figure 4 suggests that as a child's stay in an initial placement (or early in custody placement) lengthens, the likelihood that the child will receive services increases. Thus, anything that can be done to increase the likelihood that a child's placement remains stable may function as a system level intervention by decreasing system reactivity and increasing the likelihood of the provision of services to the child.

One implication of these findings is the urgency of providing intensive interventions very early in custody to deal with internalizing and/or externalizing problems. Children with more severe internalizing or externalizing problems should be provided these intervention services at the point of entry into custody. If these interventions are effective in decreasing problematic behaviors exhibited by the child, system reactivity would be expected to decrease and the child would be more likely to experience a stable placement and appropriate services. The effective use of such entry interventions implies, of course, accurate differential diagnosis and assessment at the point of entry into custody as well as the availability of the appropriate intervention technology.

Another implication of the above results concerns the need for service providers to pay attention to characteristics of the service system in which they serve clients. Characteristics of service systems clearly impact the outcomes of services (Glisson, 1994; Glisson & Hemmelgarn, 1998). As a result, clinical effectiveness research in the field would benefit from including system level variables in evaluations of clinical interventions. This is important because these and other findings show that service system characteristics may interact with intervention procedures to moderate outcomes for children.

Finally, the above results suggest that for a given level of system reactivity minority children are more likely than non-minority children to be rejected by service providers and, if services are provided, to be served farther from their home community. The reason for this is unclear. Perhaps identical problematic behaviors of minority and non-minority children are interpreted differentially. If a behavior problem exhibited by a minority child were interpreted to be a more severe problem than the same behavior problem exhibited by a non-minority child, then service providers might be more likely to reject the child and caseworkers might have greater difficulty securing mental health services for the minority child. These and earlier findings indicate that future research would benefit from further examination of the factors that contribute to reactivity versus responsiveness in children's service systems.

REFERENCES

Achenbach, T. M. (1991a). *Manual for the Child Behavior Checklist/4-18 and 1991 profile*. Burlington, VT: University of Vermont Department of Psychiatry.

Achenbach, T. M. (1991b). *Manual for the teacher's report form and 1991 profile*. Burlington, VT: University of Vermont Department of Psychiatry.

Alessi, N. E. & Magen, J. (1988). Comorbidity of other psychiatric disturbances in depressed, psychiatrically hospitalized children. *American Journal of Psychiatry, 145*, 1582-1584.

Anderson, J. C., Williams, S., McGee, R., & Silva, P. A. (1987). DSM-III disorders in preadolescent children: Prevalence in a large sample from the general population. *Archives of General Psychiatry, 44*, 69-76.

Barth, R. P., Courtney, M., Berrick, J. D., & Albert, V. (1994). *From child abuse to permanency planning*. New York: Aldine de Gruyter.

Behar, L. (1985). Changing patterns of state responsibility: A case study of North Carolina. *Journal of Clinical Child Psychology, 14*, 188-95.

Bernstein, G. A., & Borchardt, C. M. (1991). Anxiety disorders of childhood and adolescence: A critical review. *Journal of the American Academy of Child and Adolescent Psychiatry, 30*, 519-532.

Byrne, B. M. (1995). One application of structural equation modeling from two perspectives. In R. H. Hoyle (Ed.), *Structural equation modeling* (pp. 138-157). Thousand Oaks, CA: Sage.

Center for the Study of Social Policy. (1990). *The crisis in foster care: Directions for the 1990s*. Washington, DC: Center for the Study of Social Policy.

Center for the Study of Social Policy. (1993). *Kids count data book*. Washington, DC: Center for the Study of Social Policy.

Curry, J., Pelissier, B., Woodford, D., & Lockman, J. (1988). Violent or assaultive youth: Dimensional and categorical comparisons with mental health samples. *Journal of American Academy of Child and Adolescent Psychiatry, 27*, 226-232.

Dougherty, D. M., Saxe, L. M., Cross, T., & Silverman, N. (1987). *Children's mental health: Problems and services*. Durham, NC: Duke University Press.

Duchnowski, A. J., & Friedman, R. M. (1990). Children's mental health: Challenges for the nineties. *Journal of Mental Health Administration, 17*(1), 3-12.

Elliott, D. S., Huizinga, D., & Menard, S. (1989). *Multiple problem youth: Delinquency, substance use, and mental health problems*. New York, NY: Springer-Verlag.

Frank, G. (1980). Treatment needs of children in foster care. *American Journal of Orthopsychiatry, 50*(2), 256-263.

Glisson, C. (1994). The effect of services coordination teams on outcomes for children in state custody. *Administration in Social Work, 18*, 1-23.

Glisson, C. (1996). Judicial and service decisions for children entering state custody: The limited role of mental health. *Social Service Review, 70*(2), 257-81.

Glisson, C., & Hemmelgarn, A. (1998). The effects of organizational climate and interorganizational coordination on the quality and outcomes of children's service systems. *Child Abuse and Neglect, 22*(5).

Glisson, C., & James, L. (1992). The interorganizational coordination of services to children in state custody. *Administration in Social Work, 16*, 65-80.

Harrington, R., Fudge, H., Rutter, M., Pickles, A., & Hill, J. (1991). Adult outcomes of childhood and adolescent depression: II. Links with antisocial disorders. *Journal of the American Academy of Child and Adolescent Psychiatry, 30*, 434-439.

Hayduk, L. A. (1987). *Structural equation modeling with LISREL*. Baltimore, MD: The Johns Hopkins University Press.

Henggeler, S. W. (1994). A consensus: Conclusions of the APA Task Force Report on innovative models of mental health service for children, adolescents and their families. *Journal of Clinical Child Psychology, 23*(Suppl.), 3-6.

Hoyl, R., & Panter, A. (1995). Writing about structural equation models. In R. Panter, (Ed.), *Structural equation modeling: Concepts, issues, and applications*. Thousand Oaks, CA: Sage.

Joreskog, K. G., & Sorbom, D. (1993a). *LISREL 8: Structural equation modeling with the SIMPLIS command language*. Chicago: Scientific Software.

Joreskog, K. G., & Sorbom, D. (1993b). *LISREL 8: User's reference guide*. Chicago: Scientific Software.

Kahn, A. J., & Kamerman, S. B. (1992). *Integrating services integration: An overview of initiatives, issues and possibilities*. New York: National Center for Children in Poverty.

Kashani, J.H., Carlson, G.A., Beck, N.C., Hoeper, E.W., Corcoran, C.M., McAllister, J.A., Fallahi, C., Rosenberg, T.K., & Reid, J.C. (1987). Depression, depressive symptoms, and depressed mood among a community sample of adolescents. *American Journal of Psychiatry, 144*, 931-934.

Kazdin, A. E. (1995). *Conduct disorders in childhood and adolescence* (2nd ed.). Beverly Hills, CA: Sage.

King, N. J., Gullone, E., & Ollendick, T. H. (1990). Childhood anxiety disorders and depression: Phenomenology, comorbidity, and intervention issues. *Scandinavian Journal of Behaviour Therapy, 19*, 59-70.

Knitzer, J., & Yelton, S. (1990). Collaborations between child welfare and mental health. *Public Welfare, 48*, 24-33.

Kovacs, M. (1989). Affective disorders in children and adolescents. *American Psychologist, 44*(2), 209-215.

Kovacs, M., Paulauskas, S. L., Gatsonis, C., & Richards, C. (1988). Depressive disorders in childhood: III. A longitudinal study of comorbidity with and risk for conduct disorders. *Journal of Affective Disorders, 15*, 205-217.

Kovacs, M., Feinberg, T., Crouse-Novak, M., Paulauskas, S., & Finkelstein, R. (1984). Depressive disorders in childhood: I. A longitudinal prospective study of characteristics and recovery. *Archives of General Psychiatry, 41*, 229-237.

Last, C. G., Perrin, S., Hersen, M., & Kazdin, A. E. (1992). DSM-III-R anxiety disorders in children: Sociodemographic and clinical characteristics. *Journal of the American Academy of Child and Adolescent Psychiatry, 31*, 1070-1076.

Lindsey, D. (1994). *The welfare of children*. New York: Oxford University Press.

Marriage, K., Fine, S., Maretti, M., & Haley, G. (1986). Relationship between depression and conduct disorder in children and adolescents. *Journal of the American Academy of Child Psychiatry, 25*, 687-691.

McMahon, R. J. (1994). Diagnosis, assessment, and treatment of externalizing problems in children: The role of longitudinal data. Special Section: Childhood psychopathology. *Journal of Consulting and Clinical Psychology, 62*(5), 901-917.

National Advisory Mental Health Council. (1990). *National plan for research on child and adolescent mental disorders.* Rockville, MD: NIMH.

National Center on Child Abuse and Neglect (1996). *Child maltreatment 1994: Reports from the states to the National Center on Child Abuse and Neglect.* Washington, D.C.: U.S. Government Printing Office.

Nugent, W., Bruley, C., & Allen, P. (1998). The effects of aggression replacement training on antisocial behavior in a runaway shelter. *Research on Social Work Practice,* in press.

Ollendick, T. H., & King, N. J. (1994). Diagnosis, assessment, and treatment of internalizing problems in children: The role of longitudinal data. *Journal of Consulting and Clinical Psychology, 62,* 918-927.

Rosenblatt, A., & Attkinson, C. C. (1992). Integrating systems of care in California for youth with severe emotional disturbance. *Journal of Child and Family Studies, 1,* 93-113.

Rosenfeld, A. A., Pilowsky, D. J., Fine, P., Thorpe, M., Fein, E., Simms, M. D., Halfon, N., Irwin, M., Alfaro, J., Saletsky, R., & Nickman, S. (1997). Foster care: An update. *Journal of American Academy of Child and Adolescent Psychiatry, 36*(4), 448-457.

Ryan, N. D., Puig-Antich, J., Ambrosini, P., Rabinovich, H., Robinson, D., Nelson, B., Iyengar, S., & Twomey, J. (1987). The clinical picture of major depression in children and adolescents. *Archives of General Psychiatry, 44,* 854-861.

Schorr, L. B. (1997). *Common purpose: Strengthening families and neighborhoods to rebuild America.* New York: Doubleday.

Stroul, B. A. & Friedman, R. M. (1996). The system of care concept and philosophy. In B.A. Stroul (Ed.), *Children's mental health: Creating systems of care in a changing society* (pp. 3-22). Baltimore: Paul H. Brookes.

Thompson, R. A., & Wilcox, B. L. (1995). Child maltreatment research: Federal support and policy issues. *American Psychologist, 50,* 789-793.

Tuma, J. M. (1989). Mental health services for children: The state of the art. Special Issue: Children and their development: Knowledge base, research agenda, and social policy application. *American Psychologist, 44*(2), 188-199.

Webster's II New Riverside University Dictionary. (1984). Boston, MA: Riverside Publishing Co.

Webster's Ninth New Collegiate Dictionary. (1990). Springfield, MA: Merriam-Webster.

Weisz, J. R., Weersing, V. R., & Valeri, S. M. (1997). How effective is psychotherapy for children and adolescents? *Harvard Mental Health Letter, 13,* 8, February 1997.

Williams, L. J. (1996). Causal models for organizational research. Paper presented at the Children's Mental Health Services Research Center, Knoxville, TN.

The Dynamics
of Interagency Collaboration:
How Linkages Develop for Child Welfare
and Juvenile Justice Sectors
in a System of Care Demonstration

Jeanne C. Rivard
Matthew C. Johnsen
Joseph P. Morrissey
Barbara E. Starrett

SUMMARY. This paper describes results of a secondary analysis of interorganizational network data collected in an evaluation of a system-level intervention that was designed to integrate service delivery across multiple sectors serving children with serious emotional disturbances. Data measuring the extent of interorganizational resource exchange were analyzed to investigate changes in patterns of interagency collaboration involving child welfare and juvenile justice sectors. A general

---

Jeanne C. Rivard is Assistant Professor at Columbia University School of Social Work, 622 West 113th Street, New York, NY 10025. Matthew C. Johnsen is affiliated with R.O.W. Sciences, Inc., 1700 Research Boulevard, Suite 400, Rockville, MD 20850-3142. Joseph P. Morrissey and Barbara E. Starrett are affiliated with Cecil G. Sheps Center for Health Services Research, CB# 7590, 725 Airport Road, University of North Carolina at Chapel Hill, Chapel Hill, NC 27599-7590.

Address correspondence to: Jeanne Rivard, Columbia University School of Social Work, 622 West 113th Street, New York, NY 10025.

The authors wish to acknowledge the assistance of Michael O. Calloway, PhD, in reviewing earlier drafts of this paper and contributing helpful suggestions.

[Haworth co-indexing entry note]: "The Dynamics of Interagency Collaboration: How Linkages Develop for Child Welfare and Juvenile Justice Sectors in a System of Care Demonstration." Rivard, Jeanne C. et al. Co-published simultaneously in *Journal of Social Service Research* (The Haworth Press, Inc.) Vol. 25, No. 3, 1999, pp. 61-82; and: *Mental Health Services and Sectors of Care* (ed: Enola K. Proctor, Nancy Morrow-Howell, and Arlene Stiffman) The Haworth Press, Inc., 1999, pp. 61-82. Single or multiple copies of this article are available for a fee from The Haworth Document Delivery Service [1-800-342-9678, 9:00 a.m. - 5:00 p.m. (EST). E-mail address: getinfo@haworthpressinc.com].

pattern of increasing resource exchanges over time is characterized as relatively modest but important in demonstrating incremental growth in cooperative interorganizational relationships. Findings are consistent with reports documenting the project's implementation and qualitative impressions of agency respondents. *[Article copies available for a fee from The Haworth Document Delivery Service: 1-800-342-9678. E-mail address: getinfo@haworthpressinc.com]*

KEYWORDS. Child welfare, interagency collaboration, interorganizational relations, juvenile justice, network analysis, serious emotional disturbance, service sectors, system of care

For three decades, advocates and policy analysts have called for a collaborative approach on the part of child mental health, child welfare, juvenile justice, education, and health care sectors to overcome fragmentation in service delivery for children with serious emotional disturbances (Institute of Medicine, 1989; Joint Commission on the Mental Health of Children, 1969; Knitzer, 1982; National Mental Health Association, 1989; President's Commission on Mental Health, 1978; US Congress, Office of Technology Assessment, 1986). Stimulated by policy reforms, redirected public and private funding, and technical assistance, many states have demonstrated local or statewide "systems of care" (Knitzer, 1993; Lourie, Katz-Leavy, DeCarolis, & Quinlan, 1996; Rog, 1995; Stroul & Friedman, 1986). A primary objective of these systems is to develop a comprehensive array of community-based services within a collaborative infrastructure for planning, funding, developing, and delivering services. Such initiatives are intended to benefit children and families by closing gaps in the existing service delivery system, facilitating access to needed treatment and services, providing continuity of care, and increasing the likelihood of positive child and family outcomes (Attkisson, Dresser, & Rosenblatt, 1995; England & Cole, 1995; Stroul, McCormack, & Zaro, 1996).

In that a basic assumption of the system of care approach rests on the need to build a collaborative infrastructure, an important question centers on how services become integrated and how barriers, posed by fragmented organization of service delivery systems, are overcome (Sondheimer & Evans, 1995). Interorganizational theory and research have informed the measurement of system integration by providing a framework for studying relations among service organizations, emerging network structures, and factors influencing collaboration and network development (Morrissey, Johnsen, & Calloway, 1997b). In keeping with the interorganizational research tradition, this paper describes results of a secondary analysis of network data examining the development of cross-sector collaboration within a system of care demonstration for children with serious emotional disturbances in North Carolina. The study focuses directly on how interagency linkages, involving child welfare and juvenile justice organizations, develop within a system of care demonstration.

The importance of focusing on the subset of child welfare and juvenile justice agencies is evident in the literature concerning the mental health needs of children involved with child welfare (Frank, 1980; Glisson & James, 1992; Goerge, Voorhis, Grant, Casey, & Robinson, 1992; Klee & Halfon, 1987) or juvenile justice systems (Institute of Medicine, 1989). Calls within these fields urge integration of their service delivery efforts with mental health agencies (Kamerman & Kahn, 1990; Maloy, 1995). Advocates of cross-sector programming in child welfare, juvenile justice, and mental health emphasize the similarities in the characteristics of children and families served in these sectors, and argue that the door through which clients enter the service delivery system should not limit access to comprehensive service and treatment (Burns & Friedman, 1990; Glisson, 1994; Knitzer & Yelton, 1990; Robison & Binder, 1993). Studies profiling the characteristics and multi-sector service needs of children with emotional disturbances have drawn attention to the relatively high numbers of children served in child welfare and juvenile justice sectors (Polivka & Clark, 1994; Segal, 1992). A national study of 812 children with serious emotional disturbances found that child welfare services were utilized by 80% of the sample and juvenile justice services were utilized by 70.9% at some point during a seven year study period (Greenbaum, Dedrick, Friedman, Kutash, Brown, Lardieri, & Pugh, 1996).

Special efforts have been made to strengthen interactions between child welfare and mental health organizations by the National Association of Public Child Welfare Administrators and by the State Mental Health Representatives for Children and Youth, a state advocacy organization (Weber & Yelton, 1996). These efforts are motivated by the overlap in statutory requirements related to treatment and service provision; the possible benefits of sharing program and funding resources; the association between child abuse and risk of mental disorder (Kashani, Shekim, Burk, & Beck, 1987); consumer and funding source demands for less bureaucratic, efficient use of resources; and similar mandates to decrease costly out of home placements (Knitzer & Yelton, 1990; Weber & Yelton, 1996). Maloy (1995) points to the importance of fully involving the juvenile justice sector in collaborative service system development because of the juvenile courts' authority in adjudicating and determining placements for youthful offenders with serious emotional disturbances.

The setting for the analysis described here was a demonstration project that specifically targeted, among others, children with serious emotional disturbances dually served by mental health and the child welfare or juvenile justice sectors in North Carolina (Behar, 1995). The Children's Initiative in North Carolina was one of eight demonstration sites funded by the Robert Wood Johnson Foundation's Mental Health Services Program for Youth (England & Cole, 1995) to demonstrate the feasibility and effectiveness of integrating services across public child service agencies (Saxe, Cross, Lovas, & Gardner, 1995). The intervention components designed to promote local services integration will be described later in the paper.

THEORY AND RESEARCH BASE

Interorganizational theories of resource exchange and resource dependence posit that interdependencies form between organizations where there is exchange of vital organizational resources such as funding, information, and client referrals (Levine and White, 1961; Pfeffer & Salancik, 1978). Van de Ven and Ferry's model (1980) on the emergence and growth of interorganizational relationships over time emphasizes that these interdependencies grow incrementally as they are stimulated by communication, awareness of the problems faced by agencies, consensus and joint action to address problems, and structural adaptations to facilitate resource exchange and joint activities. Ring and Van de Ven (1994) suggest further that managing the development of cooperative interorganizational relationships is the key to successful joint ventures. They propose a process framework that features cyclical stages of negotiating expectations, making commitments, and executing plans. At each stage, decisions to continue or expand the collaboration are made based on assessments of the efficiency and equity of transactions. Inherent within Ring and Van de Ven's process model is the concept that individuals, within their organizational roles, affect the development of interagency relationships through establishing both professional and personal ties. This dual basis of exchange promotes trust, facilitates conflict resolution, and expedites formal and informal agreements.

Social network analysis has become a popular way to study interagency relationships. An assumption within network analysis is that patterns of interactions among service organizations can be analyzed to reveal the nature and extent of collaboration and integration within a network of service organizations (Morrissey et al., 1997b). Core variables studied in network analysis are the relations between and among organizations. The relations studied are primarily those involving the exchange of resources such as clients, funds, and information. These may be measured by type, frequency, intensity, or direction.

Considerable prior research has been conducted on the North Carolina Children's Initiative (Burns, Farmer, Angold, Costello, & Behar, 1996; John-

a total of 252 possible interorganizational ties (4 subunits by 63 organizations).

Because organizations were asked about both sending and receiving referrals and information, a confirming procedure was used to reconcile discrepant responses. Through this process, if one organization reported sending referrals to another agency, but this was not acknowledged by the other agency as being received, that response was scored as a zero value. If sending/receiving interactions were acknowledged but at differing values, the values were averaged. In that the analysis questions were aimed at comparing frequencies of interorganizational linkages at Wave I and Wave II, the valued data (0-4) were dichotomized. Zero ratings were retained as 0, but values greater than 0 were set to 1.

Data were analyzed using UCINET IV, 1.0 network analysis software (Borgatti, Everett, & Freeman, 1992), and SPSS for Windows, Release 6.0 (Norusis/SPSS Inc., 1993). Frequencies of the two types of resource exchanges at Wave I and Wave II of data collection were calculated and differences in the proportion of resource exchanges over time were tested using chi square statistics. Next, change in specific pairs of organizations was examined to determine whether the focal organizations tended to gain, lose, or maintain linkages over time. Here, the McNemar test was used to test for significance differences in interaction patterns between pairs of organizations. The McNemar test for correlated proportions, a variation of the chi square test, sets up 2 × 2 contingency tables in which the 63 pairs of interactions are assigned into one of four cells: (a) stable ties existed at both Wave I and II, (b) ties were lost at Wave II, (c) ties were gained at Wave II, and (d) no ties existed at Waves I and II (Figure 1). The McNemar procedure tests the null hypothesis that the paired proportions of the discordant cells (b and c) will be equal (Dawson-Saunders & Trapp, 1994, p. 155). This test has been utilized previously to provide a test of the significance of change within interorganizational networks (Calloway, 1993). For this study, the null hypothesis posits that there will be no difference between the number of paired linkages gained or lost over time. Increased interagency collaboration would be seen in interactions changing from no ties existing at Wave I to ties existing at Wave II (cell c).

RESULTS

Changes in Overall Patterns of Linkages

Changes in the overall pattern of linkages are based on the proportion of all possible linkages between child welfare and juvenile justice organizations

FIGURE 1. Example of Contingency Table Showing Four Categories of Change

Linkages Existing at Wave II

		Yes	No
		A	**B**
Linkages Existing at Wave I	Yes	Stable Ties	Lost Ties
		C	**D**
	No	Gained Ties	No Ties

and all other organizations in the service system. Figures 2 and 3 present the proportions of client referral and information exchanges that were reported between organizations at Waves I and II. Both figures reveal a pattern of increasing interorganizational linkages over time. The size of the increase in client referrals (Figure 2) is generally small (less than 10%), but there is a statistically significant increase in receipt of referrals by the rural child welfare organizations ($\chi^2 = 5.21$, 1 df, $p < .05$). Although more exchanges occurred at Wave II, the proportionate distribution across sectors remained fairly consistent with the pattern at Wave I. Both child welfare and juvenile justice organizations tended to send more referrals than they received, in order to access services for children and youth with serious emotional disturbances.

For information exchanges at Waves I and II (Figure 3), the rural child welfare and juvenile justice organizations fit the general pattern of small increases over time, but no change is observed for the urban child welfare organizations. However, only the change in sending information by juvenile justice organizations is significant ($\chi^2 = 3.71$, 1 df, $p = .05$).

Changes in Specific Paired Linkages

Specific pair-wise relationships were examined next to identify where most of the change was occurring within the overall pattern of increases in proportions. Tables 1 and 2 present the distribution of paired client referral exchanges and information exchanges over time within the four categories of change previously described–stable ties, lost ties, gained ties, or no ties. The

FIGURE 2. Changes in the Proportion of Client Referrals at Wave I and Wave II

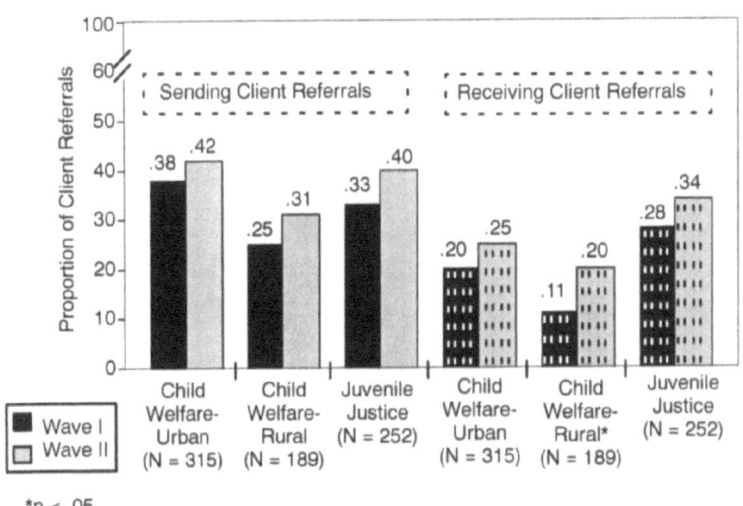

*p < .05

largest category, across sending and receiving ties for both types of resource exchanges, is the one showing no ties at Wave I and Wave II and ranges between 43% and 78% of all possible paired linkages. The large number of unconnected agencies at both time periods is due largely to the fact that these are county-based service systems and most ties occur within rather than between counties. Stable ties range between 9% and 30% of all possible linkages across referral and information networks; lost ties range between 2% and 12%; and gained ties range between 11% and 16%.

For this analysis, attention is drawn to the category of gains in linkage formation. Results of the McNemar test (Tables 1 and 2) show that a statistically significant number of new linkages were made by the rural child welfare organizations in receiving referrals ($p < .01$) and sending information ($p < .05$). The juvenile justice organizations gained a statistically significant number of new linkages through sending referrals and both sending and receiving information ($p < .05$).

The McNemar test was also conducted for each focal organization within the three main organization sets to identify whether particular functional subunits accounted for these significant gains. Within rural child welfare departments, the foster care unit produced the significant gains in referral linkages. However, the significant gains in information linkages could not be

FIGURE 3. Changes in the Proportion of Information Exchanges at Wave I and Wave II

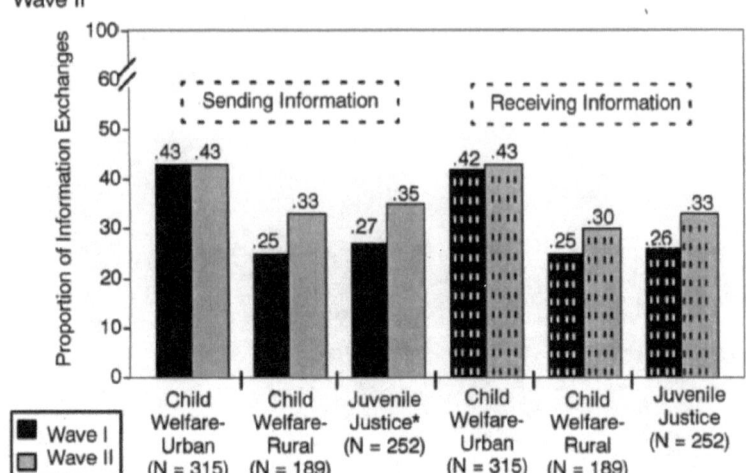

*p < .05

attributed to a single organizational unit within the rural child welfare department. The juvenile justice sector gains were due to increased resource exchanges on the part of both the juvenile evaluation center and the juvenile detention center.

Although statistically significant gains were not observed for the urban child welfare organizations as a whole, significant increases in referral exchanges were found for the child welfare intake and treatment units. However, there was a significant *decrease* in referrals for the investigations unit. In contrast to the rural child welfare department, the urban child welfare department had separate units for intake and treatment. Increases in referrals for the intake and treatment units within the urban child welfare sector might be seen to roughly parallel the increase in referrals for the rural child welfare foster care unit where intake and treatment functions were unified.

Paired interactions were further explored to discover between which organizations and sectors new linkages had formed. Table 3 presents a grid which illustrates the new linkages that formed by Wave II for the focal organizations where significant gains were found in the earlier analysis. The first column includes all organizations in the urban and the rural county, but collapses them by service sector and, in some cases, by type of service (e.g., psychiatric hospitals, residential group care, or treatment foster care). Each cell contains

TABLE 1. Distribution of Paired Client Referral Exchanges Over Time

	Number of Ties Sent				Number of Ties Received			
	Stable ties at Waves I and II	Lost ties by Wave II	Gained ties by Wave II	No ties at Waves I and II	Stable ties at Waves I and II	Lost ties by Wave II	Gained ties by Wave II	No ties at Waves I and II
Urban Child Welfare (N = 315)	81	39	50	145	35	28	45	207
Rural Child Welfare (N = 189)	32	15	27	115	17	4	20**	148
Juvenile Justice (N = 252)	61	21	39*	131	50	20	35	147

* $p < .05$
** $p < .01$

the type of linkage that was formed by each focal organization. A linkage was recorded in the table if it occurred between the focal organization and one or more organizations within a specified sector.

Table 3 shows that the new linkages formed by child welfare and juvenile justice organizations ranged across most service sectors. New ties within the child welfare sector (e.g., ties between the rural foster unit and other child welfare organizations) and within the juvenile justice sector mean that linkages were expanded between various functional units within these sectors. Although not indicated on the table, many new linkages were made across counties suggesting greater regional collaboration. Table 3 shows the juvenile evaluation center to have made the largest gains in forging both types of linkages across nearly all sectors in the service system.

Fewer new ties were created with special education and health care sectors. A review of the data showed that information linkages with special education tended to be stable over time (i.e., exist at both Waves I and II). Further analysis of stable ties and lost ties is certainly warranted and will be explored in future analyses.

TABLE 2. Distribution of Paired Information Exchanges Over Time

	Number of Ties Sent				Number of Ties Received			
	Stable ties at Waves I and II	Lost ties by Wave II	Gained ties by Wave II	No ties at Waves I and II	Stable ties at Waves I and II	Lost ties by Wave II	Gained ties by Wave II	No ties at Waves I and II
Urban Child Welfare (N = 315)	95	42	41	137	96	36	38	145
Rural Child Welfare (N = 189)	33	15	29*	112	29	18	28	114
Juvenile Justice (N = 252)	55	13	33*	151	52	14	31*	155

* $p < .05$

Progress Reports and Qualitative Impressions of Project Implementation

Following the planning year, the Children's Initiative was granted four years of funding to carry out their plans and reach their goals. The data used in the present secondary analysis was collected at the end of the first year of implementation in 1991 and at the end of the third year in 1993. Progress reports detailing how objectives were achieved through the end of the third year of implementation illustrate service development activities that specifically involved child welfare and juvenile justice or impacted their clients (NCDHR, 1991, 1992, 1993). These included: (a) the addition or expansion of case management services, in-home intervention, treatment foster care, high management group homes, respite, and crisis stabilization; (b) joint funding and programming between area mental health programs and county departments of social services for services most needed by child welfare clients including emergency respite and crisis stabilization; (c) joint planning with social services and child welfare to move toward pooled funding via the development of client information tracking systems and expanding foster care funding to finance residential treatment costs; (d) expanding Medicaid coverage to finance community-based treatment; (e) on-site provision of youthful sex offender treatment program and substance abuse services by

TABLE 3. Types of New Interorganizational Linkages Formed Between Child Welfare and Juvenile Justice Focal Organizations and Other Service Sectors

ALL SERVICE SECTORS	CHILD WELFARE			JUVENILE JUSTICE	
	Rural Foster Care	**Urban Intake**	**Urban Treatment**	**Detention Center**	**Evaluation Center**
Mental Health Center	Referral Information	Referral	Referral	Information	Referral Information
Child Welfare	Referral Information	Referral	Referral	Information	Referral Information
Juvenile Justice	Referral	Referral	---	Information	Referral Information
Special Education	---	---	Referral	---	Information
Health Care	Information	---	---	---	---
Psychiatric Hospital	Referral Information	Referral	Referral	---	Referral Information
Residential Group Care or TFC	Referral Information	Referral	Referral	Information	Referral Information
Other Family and Social Services	---	Referral	Referral	Information	Referral Information
Advocacy and Training	---	Referral	Referral	---	---
Police and Sheriff	---	---	Referral	Information	Referral Information

Referral = New linkages formed by Wave II through sending or receiving client referrals
Information = New linkages formed by Wave II through sending or receiving information

area mental health counselors at the juvenile evaluation center, and expansion of case management for the substance abuse unit; and (f) development of a formal protocol guiding interagency team functioning and plans to disseminate the protocol through training.

Review of responses to open-ended questions illustrate child welfare and juvenile justice team members' perspectives of the developing service system. Organizations which showed gains in resource exchanges expressed high levels of involvement on project management teams, interagency councils, and treatment teams. Some respondents commented on having been involved in the initial project planning phases. This initial investment appeared to offset the difficulties encountered in the collaboration process. With regard to changes in services and programs, representatives from both child welfare and juvenile justice remarked on the new services available. However, it was also clear that new pressures were bearing down on agencies in the form of: more children entering foster care, more dysfunctional and hard-to-place children presenting for service, and more serious and violent delinquents requiring a range of services. When asked about how the current service system performs in meeting the needs of youth, respondents generally noted improvement in the system but stressed that many needs remained unmet including: waiting lists for services; lack of adequate numbers of residential and respite placements; lack of transition services for older youths; difficulties in obtaining services for certain groups of youths such as sex offenders, black males, homeless youth, and those who did not qualify for the project.

Several respondents commented that the interagency councils were beneficial in distributing responsibility for children's care among agencies and in promoting communication and cooperation. Others commented that some confusion remained about the goals of the project and that there were unmet expectations regarding service development. The effects of the child-specific treatment teams seemed more visible to respondents. Overwhelmingly, the sentiments expressed were positive, but several respondents noted that the effectiveness of the treatment teams varied due to personalities, leadership, and disputes over the best interests of the child versus agency priorities. A newly developed interagency teamwork protocol was mentioned several times as being very helpful in clarifying roles and distributing decision-making.

DISCUSSION

The "system of care" model (Stroul & Friedman, 1986) presumes the formation of new partnerships among major service sectors as a result of interventions that provide opportunities for collaboration at administrative and direct service levels. By examining the growth in connectedness of child welfare and juvenile justice organizations within the service network, we found evidence of incremental growth in partnerships that supports the system of care model as well as the frameworks proposed by Van de Ven and Ferry (1980) and Ring and Van de Ven (1994). The multi-level governance structure established during the planning stage shows that a strong foundation was laid through communicating and reaching consensus about the need for an interagency approach to improving the service system, and about how target problems would be addressed. This groundwork corresponds to Van de Ven and Ferry's (1980) modeling of the requisite need for such consensus to stimulate resource exchange, and to Ring and Van de Ven's (1994) early negotiation and commitment stages in which the parties engage in developing joint expectations, bargaining, sense-making, and deriving formal and informal means for initiating joint action.

Tasks carried out by the various teams during the implementation phases of the project parallel Ring and Van de Ven's (1994) description of the execution stage of cooperative interorganizational relationship development in which formally assigned roles, responsibilities, and tasks are put in motion with periodic assessment and renegotiation. Their accomplishments, specifically related to meeting the service needs of children with serious emotional disturbances in the care of child welfare and juvenile justice, illustrate how critical issues (Knitzer & Yelton, 1990; Soler, 1992) pertinent to these sectors were being addressed.

The quantitative findings show a general pattern of increasing resource exchanges over time with particular growth in referral and information linkages made by juvenile justice agencies and child welfare organizational units with primary responsibilities for intake, treatment, and placement. Juvenile justice agencies made the greatest gains in establishing new linkages with organizations across all major service sectors. Growth in referral linkages initiated by the child welfare and juvenile justice sectors illustrate the development of interagency collaboration through the acquisition of needed resources for children with serious emotional disturbances. As agencies interact more through interagency forums they tend to become more aware of other services that are available to meet their clients' needs and, thus, to make more referrals. The strong growth in interagency connections observed for the juvenile justice evaluation center and detention center is seen as a promising pathway leading from institutional care to community-based care. Gains in information exchange for purposes of coordination, control, planning, or evaluation demonstrate greater investment and commitment to resolve problems and take joint action. Though there were significant increases in interagency connections over time, the gains are characterized as relatively modest but important in demonstrating incremental growth in cooperative interorganizational relationships. These findings are consistent with qualitative impressions of agency representatives who acknowledged the growth in interagency relations, but stressed the need for improved structuring of interagency team processes and the need to see a return on their interagency investments in the form of service resources for their clients.

There are two main limitations to this study. First, because data were collected at the end of the first year of program implementation, the absence of a true baseline in the current study may underestimate the change that occurred and can be attributed to the demonstration. Second, by focusing only on the 63 organizations present at both Wave I and Wave II, the present analysis underestimates the total amount of change. In some cases, new organizations and organizational "units" were created in response to intervention efforts and in other instances, they were established by existing agencies in an effort to fill service gaps. In both cases, the system of care may have been expanded in important ways not considered in the present analysis. However, this organizational set analysis was conducted to specifically examine change in interorganizational relationships between organizations existing at both time periods which had been exposed to the intervention. Changes in the service system as a whole, including new organizations established by Wave II, are reported by Johnsen and colleagues (1996) and Morrissey and colleagues (1997a).

In conclusion, child welfare and juvenile justice agencies stand on the front line in serving the most troubled children and families. The large number of children entering their systems and their dual custodial and treatment responsibilities necessitate their involvement as central players in collaborative initiatives, and also place them in a pivotal position to influence the growth and development of systems of care. Direct implications for planning and implementing interagency projects that involve these key child service sectors emerged from the quantitative findings and review of the qualitative data and progress reports. An extended planning period with high levels of involvement by child welfare and juvenile justice provides a strong beginning and milieu for discussing motivations and joint expectations, for initial positioning and bargaining, and for setting the stage to take joint action. The multi-level team approach (client-specific, county, regional, and state) appears to distribute power and encourage ownership of the project. Built-in monitoring and problem resolution strategies ensure that issues or problems are addressed, and attention to these matters by multiple team levels prevent them from disappearing from the agenda. Planning and implementation efforts, specifically targeting the service needs of children and youth with serious emotional disturbances in the care of child welfare and juvenile justice, increases the likelihood of expanding funding and services for these youth. Findings of this analysis also highlight the need to place a greater emphasis on the developmental process issues up front. For example, it is important to clarify expectations that are critical to the continuance of the interorganizational relationship and negotiate how these will be met. One of the most valuable lessons, pertinent to the process focus, is the importance of developing an interagency teamwork protocol early in the implementation phases to facilitate the emergence of an effective team.

NOTES

1. To confirm that relevant organizations were included in the network, one of the questionnaire items asked respondents to identify all of the key people playing leadership roles in developing mental health services. A comparison of the organizational affiliations of individuals named on this item with the final list of organizations

bounded in the network showed that the only potential members of the network missing were private practitioners such as physicians, psychologists, and psychiatrists. However, individual practitioners had been deliberately excluded from the network survey which focused at the organizational level.

2. The same organizational positions were surveyed at both time periods, but individuals occupying these positions were not always the same. At the second wave of data collection, 56% of respondents were the same as Wave I. Although every attempt was made to survey the same respondents, turnover in agency personnel precluded this possibility. However, different respondents over time should not affect findings of the interorganizational network survey because respondents were asked to rate the extent of resources exchanged between their organization and all others in the present tense without regard for change which might have occurred.

3. Returning to the issue of different respondents at Waves I and II, seven of these 12 respondents were different than those surveyed at Wave I. Lack of historic perspective could affect the qualitative data because respondents were specifically asked about change in these questions. However, because the open-ended questions were more broadly focused on organizations' roles in the Children's Initiative and on the service system in general, respondents were able to reasonably answer the questions if they had historic knowledge of their organizations and experience in the service system. Review of the demographic data for these seven respondents showed they had been employed in their current positions on average 11.71 months, but had been working in the same child welfare or juvenile justice organization on average 8.67 years.

REFERENCES

Attkisson, C. C., Dresser, K. L., & Rosenblatt, A. (1995). Service systems for youth with severe emotional disorder: System-of-care research in California. In L. Bickman & D. J. Rog (Eds.), *Children's mental health services: Research, policy, and evaluation* (pp. 236-277). Thousand Oaks, CA: Sage Publications.

Behar, L. (1995). State-level policies in children's mental health: An example of system building and refinancing. In L. Bickman & D. J. Rog (Eds.), *Children's mental health services: Research, policy, and evaluation* (pp. 21-41). Thousand Oaks, CA: Sage Publications.

Borgatti, S., Everett, M., & Freeman, L. (1992). *UCINET IV, 1.0.* Columbia, SC: Analytic Technologies.

Burns, B. J., Farmer, E. M. Z., Angold, A., Costello, E. J., & Behar, L. (1996). A randomized trial of case management for youths with serious emotional disturbance. *Journal of Clinical Child Psychology, 25*(4), 476-486.

Burns, B. J., & Friedman, R. M. (1990). Examining the research base for child mental health services and policy. *Journal of Mental Health Administration, 17*(1), 87-98.

Calloway, M. O. (1993). *A method and a measure for assessing structural change in interorganizational networks.* Doctoral dissertation, Department of Sociology and Anthropology, North Carolina State University, Raleigh, NC.

Dawson-Saunders, B., & Trapp, R. G. (1994). *Basic and clinical biostatistics.* East Norwalk, CT: Appleton & Lange.

England, M. J., & Cole, R. J. (1995). Children and mental health: How can the system be improved? *Health Affairs, Fall,* 131-138.

Evan, W. M. (1976). An organization-set model of interorganizational relations. In W. M. Evan (Ed.), *Interorganizational relations* (pp.78-90). Pittsburgh, PA: University of Pennsylvania Press.

Frank, G. (1980). Treatment needs of children in foster care. *American Journal of Orthopsychiatry, 50*(2), 256-263.

Glisson, C. (1994). The effect of services coordination teams on outcomes for children in state custody. *Administration in Social Work, 18*(4), 1-23.

Glisson, C., & James, L. (1992). The interorganizational coordination of services to children in state custody. *Administration in Social Work, 16*(3/4), 65-80.

Goerge, R. M., Voorhis, J. V., Grant, S., Casey, K., & Robinson, M. (1992). Special education experiences of foster children: An empirical study. *Child Welfare, LXXI(5),* 419-437.

Greenbaum, P. E., Dedrick, R. F., Friedman, R. M., Kutash, K., Brown, E. C., Lardieri, S. P., & Pugh, A. M. (1996). National adolescent and child treatment study (NACTS): Outcomes for children with serious emotional and behavioral disturbance. *Journal of Emotional and Behavioral Disorders, 4*(3), 130-146.

Institute of Medicine (1989). *Research on children and adolescents with mental, behavioral, and developmental disorders: Mobilizing a national initiative.* Washington, DC: National Academy Press.

Johnsen, M. C., Morrissey, J. P., & Calloway, M. O. (1996). Structure and change in child mental health service delivery networks. *Journal of Community Psychology, 24*(3), 275-289.

Joint Commission on Mental Health of Children (1969). *Crisis in child mental health: Challenge for the 1970s.* New York: Harper & Row.

Kamerman, S. B., & Kahn, A. J. (1990). Social services for children, youth, and families in the United States. *Children & Youth Services Review, 12*(1/2), Special Issue.

Kashani, J. H., Shekim, W. O., Burk, J. P., & Beck, N. C. (1987). Abuse as a predictor of psychopathology in children and adolescents. *Journal of Clinical Child Psychology, 16,* 43-50.

Klee, L., & Halfon, N. (1987). Mental health care for foster children in California. *Child Abuse and Neglect, 11,* 63-64.

Knitzer, J. (1982). *Unclaimed children: The failure of public responsibility to children and adolescents in need of mental health services.* Washington, DC: Children's Defense Fund.

Knitzer, J. (1993). Children's mental health policy: Challenging the future. *Journal of Emotional and Behavioral Disorders, 1*(1), 8-16.

Knitzer, J., & Yelton, S. (1990). Collaborations between child welfare and mental health. *Public Welfare, Spring,* 24-33.

Levine, S., & White, P. E. (1961). Exchange as a conceptual framework for the study of interorganizational relationships. *Administrative Science Quarterly, 5,* 583-601.

Lourie, I. S., Katz-Leavy, J., DeCarolis, G., & Quinlan, W. A. (1996). The role of the federal government. In B. A. Stroul (Ed.), *Children's mental health: Creating systems of care in a changing society* (pp. 99-114). Baltimore, MD: Paul H. Brookes Publishing Co.

Maloy, K. A. (1995). Juvenile justice: Once and future gatekeeper for a system of care. In L. Bickman & D.J. Rog (Eds.), *Children's mental health services: Research, policy, and evaluation* (pp. 171-205). Thousand Oaks, CA: Sage Publications, Inc.

Morrissey, J. P. (1992). An interorganizational network approach to evaluating children's mental health service systems. In L. Bickman & D. J. Rog (Eds.), *New directions for program evaluation* (Vol. 54, pp. 85-98). San Francisco, CA: Jossey-Bass.

Morrissey, J. P., Johnsen, M. C., & Calloway, M. O. (1997a). Evaluating performance and change in mental health systems serving children and youth: An interorganizational network approach. *Journal of Mental Health Administration, 24*(1), 4-22.

Morrissey, J. P., Johnsen, M. C., & Calloway, M. O. (1997b). Methods for system-level evaluations of child mental health service networks. In M. Epstein, K. Kutash, & A. Duchnowski (Eds.), *Community based programming for children with serious emotional disturbance and the families: Research and evaluations.* Austin, TX: PRO-ED, Inc.

National Mental Health Association (1989). *Report of the Invisible Children Project.* Author.

North Carolina Department of Human Resources Division of Mental Health, Developmental Disabilities, and Substance Abuse Services. (1990). *North Carolina Mental Health Services Program for Youth.* Raleigh, NC: Author.

North Carolina Department of Human Resources Division of Mental Health, Developmental Disabilities, and Substance Abuse Services. (1991) *North Carolina's Mental Health Services Program for Youth: Annual report to Robert Wood Johnson Foundation-Year 1.* Raleigh, NC: Author.

North Carolina Department of Human Resources Division of Mental Health, Developmental Disabilities, and Substance Abuse Services. (1992). *North Carolina's Mental Health Services Program for Youth: The Children's Initiative-Reapplication proposal to Robert Wood Johnson Foundation.* Raleigh, NC: Author.

North Carolina Department of Human Resources Division of Mental Health, Developmental Disabilities, and Substance Abuse Services. (1993). *North Carolina's Mental Health Services Program for Youth: Annual report to Robert Wood Johnson Foundation-Year 3.* Raleigh, NC: Author.

Norusis, M. J., & SPSS Inc. (1993). *SPSS for Windows Release 6.0.* Chicago, IL: SPSS.

Pfeffer, J., & Salancik, G. R. (1978). *The external control of organizations: A resource dependence perspective.* New York: Harper and Row.

Polivka, B. J., & Clark, J. A. (1994). A collaborative system of care for youth with severe emotional disturbances: An evaluation of client characteristics and services. *Journal of Mental Health Administration, 21*(2), 170-184.

President's Commission on Mental Health (1978). *Report to the president from the President's Commission on Mental Health* (Vols. 1 and 3). Washington, DC: Government Printing Office.

Ring, P. S., & Van de Ven, A. H. (1994). Developmental processes of cooperative interorganizational relationships. *Academy of Management Review, 19*(1), 90-118.

Robison, S., & Binder, H. (1993). Building bridges for families: States are filling gaps among child welfare, juvenile justice, and mental health agencies. *Public Welfare, Summer*, 15-20.

Rog, D. J. (1995). The status of children's mental health: An overview. In L. Bickman & D.J. Rog (Eds.), *Children's mental health services: Research, policy, and evaluation* (pp. 3-18). Thousand Oaks, CA: Sage Publications, Inc.

Saxe, L., Cross, T. P., Lovas, G. S., & Gardner, J. K. (1995). Evaluation of the mental health services program for youth: Examining rhetoric in action. In L. Bickman & D. J. Rog (Eds.), *Children's mental health services: Research, policy, and evaluation* (pp. 206-235). Thousand Oaks, CA: Sage Publications.

Segal, E. A. (1992). Multineed children in the social services system. *Social Work in Education, 14*(3), 190-198.

Soler, M. (1992). Interagency services in juvenile justice systems. In I. M. Schwartz (Ed.), *Juvenile justice and public policy* (pp. 134-150). New York: Lexington Books.

Sondheimer, D. L., & Evans, M. E. (1995). Developments in children's mental health services research: An overview of current and future directions. In L. Bickman & D. J. Rog (Eds.), *Children's mental health services: Research, policy, and evaluation* (pp. 64-84). Thousand Oaks, CA: Sage Publications.

Stroul, B. A., & Friedman, R. M. (1986). *A system of care for children and youth with severe emotional disturbances* (Rev. ed.). Washington, DC: Georgetown University Child Development Center, CASSP Technical Assistance Center.

Stroul, B. A., & Friedman, R. M. (1996). The system of care concept and philosophy. In B. A. Stroul (Ed.), *Children's mental health: Creating systems of care in a changing society* (pp. 3-21). Baltimore, MD: Paul H. Brookes Publishing Co.

Stroul, B. A., McCormack, M., & Zaro, S. M. (1996). Measuring outcomes in systems of care. In B. A. Stroul (Ed.), *Children's mental health: Creating systems of care in a changing society* (pp. 313-336). Baltimore, MD: Paul H. Brookes Publishing Co.

U.S. Congress Office of Technology Assessment (1986). *Children's mental health: Problems and services–A background paper*. Washington, DC: Author.

Van de Ven, A., & Ferry, D. (1980). *Measuring and assessing organizations*. New York: Wiley.

Weber, M., & Yelton, S. (1996). The role of the child welfare system in systems of care. In B. A. Stroul (Ed.), *Children's mental health: Creating systems of care in a changing society* (pp. 215-233). Baltimore, MD: Paul H. Brookes Publishing Co.

Youth and Provider Perspectives on Social Service Providers' Roles in Mental Health Services

Arlene Rubin Stiffman
Diane Elze
Eric Hadley-Ives
Sharon Johnson

SUMMARY. In 1994 and 1996, the Youth Services Project interviewed 792 youths from St. Louis City. Although the youths showed a high need for mental health services (20% met diagnostic criteria), less than half of the youths with problems received services. Past contact with a social service provider, but not a teacher, physician, etc., significantly predicted care for mental health problems (odds ratio = 1.5). Social service professionals (largely social workers) served more youths than did any other profession. Of youths with persistent problems, 25% received services from social service professionals, 3% from MD/PhD level psychiatrists or psychologists, 7% from primary care medical doctors, 12% from teachers/coaches, 15% from other helpers, and 37% received no services at all. *[Article copies available for a fee from The Haworth Document Delivery Service: 1-800-342-9678. E-mail address: getinfo@haworthpressinc.com]*

Arlene Rubin Stiffman, Diane Elze, Eric Hadley-Ives, and Sharon Johnson are affiliated with The George Warren Brown School of Social Work, Center for Mental Health Services Research, Washington University, St. Louis, MO 63130.

This research was supported by the National Institute of Mental Health Grants #R24-MH50857 and R24-MH-56425-01.

[Haworth co-indexing entry note]: "Youth and Provider Perspectives on Social Service Providers' Roles in Mental Health Services." Stiffman, Arlene Rubin et al. Co-published simultaneously in *Journal of Social Service Research* (The Haworth Press, Inc.) Vol. 25, No. 3, 1999, pp. 83-97; and: *Mental Health Services and Sectors of Care* (ed: Enola K. Proctor, Nancy Morrow-Howell, and Arlene Stiffman) The Haworth Press, Inc., 1999, pp. 83-97. Single or multiple copies of this article are available for a fee from The Haworth Document Delivery Service [1-800-342-9678, 9:00 a.m. - 5:00 p.m. (EST). E-mail address: getinfo@haworthpressinc.com].

83

KEYWORDS. Adolescents, mental health services, service pathways, mental health service providers, social service providers

This paper examines the role of social service providers in helping adolescents using public service sectors to access mental health services. Access to services is a major issue for adolescents. Although the literature shows that the need for adolescent mental health services is high (Brandenburg, Friedman & Silver, 1990; Stiffman & Cunningham, 1990), most youths with problems never access services. For example, although an estimated 14% to 25% of youths have diagnosable disorders (e.g., Burns, Costello, Angold, Tweed, Stangl, Farmer, & Erkanli, 1995; Costello, 1989; Offord, Boyle, Flemin, Blum & Rae-Grant, 1989), only 4% to 10% of youths who need services get them (e.g., Burns et al., 1995; Burns & Taube, 1989; Costello, Angold, Burns, Farmer, Stangl, Erkanli, & Messerm, 1995; Saunders, Resnick, Hoberman, & Blum, 1994).

Access to mental health services for youths largely depends on the recognition and actions of key adults (Landsverk, in press; Pescosolido, 1992; Proctor & Stiffman, 1998), as few adolescents want or seek mental health services on their own (Landsverk, in press). Typically, parents, teachers, juvenile justice authorities, or others direct youths to resources. The literature shows that youths with mental health disorders that are not troubling to adults, such as depression, are less likely to receive services (Garland, 1995) than are youths with conduct problems (Cohen, Kasen, Brook, & Struening, 1991; Earls, Robins, Stiffman et al., 1989). In the case of conduct problems, the conflict these youths have with parents and other authorities prompts the adult to seek services for the youth. Further, the few youths who receive care receive it in multiple sectors, with only 1% receiving services in the mental health sector. Most who receive care receive it through educational or primary health sectors (Costello et al., 1995), or through the child welfare or juvenile justice sectors (Stiffman, Chen, Elze, Dore & Cheng, 1997).

Given that youths infrequently seek help on their own from the mental health sector, the role of providers in accessing services has direct implications for improving the provision rates for mental health services. Mental health services research shows that providers' knowledge and awareness is as, or more, salient than need or service availability in obtaining services for teens (Costello, Burns, Costello, Edelbrock, Dulcan & Brent, 1988; Horwitz, Leaf, Leventhal, Borsyth & Speechley, 1992; Stiffman et al., 1997). Providers who might serve as gateways to services must be able to identify the youths' problems and they must know enough about services to help the youths access them. In the public sector, four types of service sectors function as gateways to the mental health sector services: child welfare, juvenile justice, primary health, and education. The role of these gateway sectors is to provide minimal auxiliary or temporary services or connections to services, not to provide inpatient or outpatient psychiatric services themselves (Lourie & Katz-Leavy, 1991). Therefore the gateway provider plays an especially key role in identifying and referring youths to appropriate help. Often he/she has the first contact with the youth, identifies the problem, provides some immediate services, and/or refers the youth to psychiatric or other direct mental health services.

Of all types of providers, social service providers (who are largely trained as social workers) are the only ones who are identified with both the specialty mental health sector and with gateway sectors (Callicutt & Lecca, 1983; Taube & Barrett, 1983; Lourie, 1987). Research on their function within the specialty mental health sector demonstrates that social workers provide as high a quality of services, as measured by consumer satisfaction (*Consumer Reports*, 1995; Seligman, 1996), as psychiatrists or psychologists. Social service providers are multi-sector providers. They function within the full range of child and adolescent specialty mental health service sectors, including private and public psychiatric hospitals and inpatient units, residential treatment centers, day treatment and partial hospitalization programs, and outpatient clinics. However, they also staff gateway sector services such as school counseling services, youth emergency shelters, crisis hotlines, community centers, drop-in centers, street outreach programs, juvenile justice services, and health care facilities.

Other providers are associated more closely with only one gateway sector. In the education sector, teachers and coaches, along with social service providers (school social workers or counselors), constitute an integral part of the education-based service delivery team, addressing a range of psychosocial issues including depression and suicidal ideation (Harold & Harold, 1993). Similarly, in the health sector, primary care physicians, along with social service providers (health social workers and counselors), serve as gateways or filters to the specialty mental health sector (Marino, Gallo, Ford, & Anthony, 1995).

In this paper, we examine the role of different providers in serving the mental health service needs of adolescents by asking four key questions. Who provides the mental health services that the youths receive? Which providers facilitate the youths' access to services? Which providers serve youths with more problems? Does the quality of services differ by type of profession?

METHODS

Design. The Youth Services Project, funded by the National Institute of Mental Health, examined adolescents' need for and use of mental health services over a two-year period. All youths were from the city of St. Louis, and recruited from health, child welfare, juvenile justice, or education sectors. All four service sectors were in a position to screen youths for mental health problems and to either provide some mental health services or refer to services elsewhere. Youths were interviewed in 1994 and re-interviewed in 1996.

Sample. The Youth Services Project recruited subjects with the aid of service providers, by having interviewers approach youths in the service sector waiting rooms, and by letters and posters requesting volunteers from each sector's service users. Unfortunately, no records were kept concerning the response rates from the varying recruitment methods. Trained professional interviewers administered individual interviews, averaging 55 minutes in length, to each respondent. The Internal Review Board at Washington University approved all methods, and the National Institute of Mental Health issued a Certificate of Confidentiality. Interviewers obtained informed consent from all subjects and their guardians. When possible, the interviewer completed the interview on site, immediately before or after services were obtained. Otherwise, the interviewer arranged an appointment for a future interview in the youth's home, or at a mutually acceptable site.

In 1994, the 792 subjects were all between 13 and 17 years of age, with a mean age of 15.3 years. Eighty-five percent were traced and re-interviewed in 1996. Thirteen percent were white, 86% Black, and 1% other. Forty-three percent were male and 57% female. The occupation of the parent who provided the most financial support to the family in the last 6 months determined the youth's socioeconomic status. Accordingly, 15% were welfare recipients, 39% laborers or semiskilled workers, 23% blue collar, 14% white collar, and 8% professional. Fifty-three percent of the children lived in families headed by a mother only, 14% in two parent families, 15% in foster or group care, 12% with nonparent relatives, and 6% elsewhere. There were no significant demographic differences between the 1994 and 1996 samples.

In order to assess the potential generalizability of the study sample to clients of each service sector, we compared the demographics of the interview sample with clinic records from the health sector and with anonymous tallies of clients from the other gateway sectors. (The other sectors kept no clinic records.) These comparisons showed that the interview sample was quite representative of adolescent clients from each sector. Youths sampled from the child welfare or educational sectors did not differ in race, gender, or age from clients of the respective public sectors. However, our health interviewees averaged three months younger than teenagers using the health sector; and our juvenile justice interviewees had fewer males (60% vs. 75%) and averaged 2 months younger than teenagers using the juvenile justice sector. Note that teenage clients from the public sectors and our interview sample are not representative of the population of St. Louis City, which is closer to 50% Black and 50% White. However, they are representative of public sector clients.

Instruments. Highly structured interview protocols yielded data concerning the youths' mental health and service use.

Mental health measures. Measures of depression, conduct disorder, and substance (alcohol and drug) abuse or dependence came from the Diagnostic Interview Schedule for Children-Revised (Cohen, Velez, Kohn, Schwab-Stone, & Johnson, 1987; Schaffer, Schwab-Stone, Fischer & Cohen, 1993). The DISC-R allows two separate operationalizations of mental health problems: (1) a diagnosis of disorder based on computer algorithms that combine symptoms according to the criteria in DSM-IV; and, (2) a count of serious symptoms (e.g., those lasting 2 weeks or more, or those that interfere significantly with the youth's life). Information about suicidality was derived from questions in the DISC Depression section that asked about thoughts of death, suicide plans, and suicide attempts in the last six months.

Service use measures. The youths' use of mental health services was broadly defined, and questions concerning use were asked in 1994 and 1996. In 1994, youths were asked if they were helped within each of the four service sectors for one of the following problems: sadness/depression, feeling suicidal, fears/stress, misbehavior/getting in trouble, alcohol or drug use, or other emotional or social problems. If they received any help, they were then asked which type of professional provided that help (psychiatrist, MD, social worker, teacher, counselor, etc.).

In 1996, we obtained information about any services received since the prior interview two years earlier. The questionnaire first asked the youths if they had received any services for emotional or behavioral problems where they stayed away from home overnight (inpatient care, foster care, group homes, emergency shelters, detention centers or prisons, summer camp programs). Then the questionnaire asked them if they had received any help through their schools (special school, special classes, special resources, counseling); or any outpatient care (community mental health centers, private practitioners, physicians); or any other help (hotlines, peer support groups). This set of questions was based upon the introductory section of the Services Assessment for Children and Adolescents (SACA) (Horwitz, Hoagwood, Stiffman et al., in preparation; Stiffman, Horwitz, Hoagwood et al., in review).

In 1996, the youths were asked details about specific providers who had helped them in the last six months. The youths were asked whether they had any contact in the last six months with each of five different sectors of care (education, health, juvenile justice, child welfare, or mental health). If they had used a sector's services, they were asked if they had spoken to anyone at that sector about each item on a list of general mental health problems. These included sadness or depression, family problems, suicidal feelings, behavior, violence, getting in other trouble, worries, fears, stress, and drug or alcohol use. Then they were asked who had helped them, the extent of that help, and how much they felt they were helped by the service (on a 3-point scale from "not at all" to "a lot").

Validation of provider professions. Youths' reports of the profession, role, and training of the provider were verified, and corrected as needed, through a survey of all those providers. In this extension study, also funded by NIMH, providers responded concerning their profession, education, training and current position. In all, we were able to verify the role of 68% (365) of the providers, contacting 62% personally. These 68% served 84% of the 281 youths' who had reported services in the six months prior to the 1996 interview. Of the 281 youths, 141 had seen multiple providers (mean = 2.1). The youths' misattribution errors for provider profession were typically small (calling a social worker a guidance counselor). These errors were made in approximately 1/3 of their attributions of provider profession. In each case, we corrected the data to correspond with the providers' reports.

Analyses. Prior to beginning data analyses, we used provider responses to classify providers into five categories. Four of these categories comprise providers who serve as gateways or filters to mental health services, and one category consists of psychiatrists or PhD level psychologists. We based this categorization on their training and role, resulting in the following categories: (1) psychiatrists and PhD level psychologists who were mental health specialists; (2) primary care MDs; (3) social service providers (25% had MSW degrees or a PhD in social work, 30% had BAs or BSWs but called themselves social workers; others were largely guidance counselors with MAs in educational psychology); (4) teachers or coaches; and (5) "other providers" (judges, nurses' aides, janitors, youth leaders, principals, etc.).

Logistic regression analyses were used to answer the question of "Which providers facilitate the youths' access to mental health services?" The regressions examined how the severity and persistence of youths' mental health problems and their earlier contact with various types of providers predicted receipt of services between 1994 and 1996. Frequency tables were used to answer the questions concerning "Who provides the mental health services that the youths receive?" and "Which providers serve youths with more problems?" Analysis of variance with post-hoc means tests address the question of "Does the quality of services differ by type of profession?" For this analysis, we used a STATA program that accounted for clustering by subject ID since youths often gave ratings for more than one type of provider (mean was 2.5 providers per youth) (StataCorp, 1997).

RESULTS

To understand the youths' need for and use of services, some background data on the youths' mental health is warranted. In both 1994 and 1996, the youths showed a high need for mental health services (20% met criteria for at least one mental health disorder, and 50% had 3 or more symptoms). These problems were often persistent: 14% (n = 95) of youths met diagnostic criteria for a disorder in both 1994 and 1996; and 31% (n = 209) displayed significant symptoms of a disorder at both interviews. However, over the two-year period, only 44% of even those youths with persistent problems (they had the same problem in both 1994 and in 1996) received any services, and even lower percentages received help specifically for that problem (Figure 1). In fact, service rates were higher for youths who only had persistent

FIGURE 1. Number of Youths with a Persistent Problem (in both 1994 and 1996) by Services Received

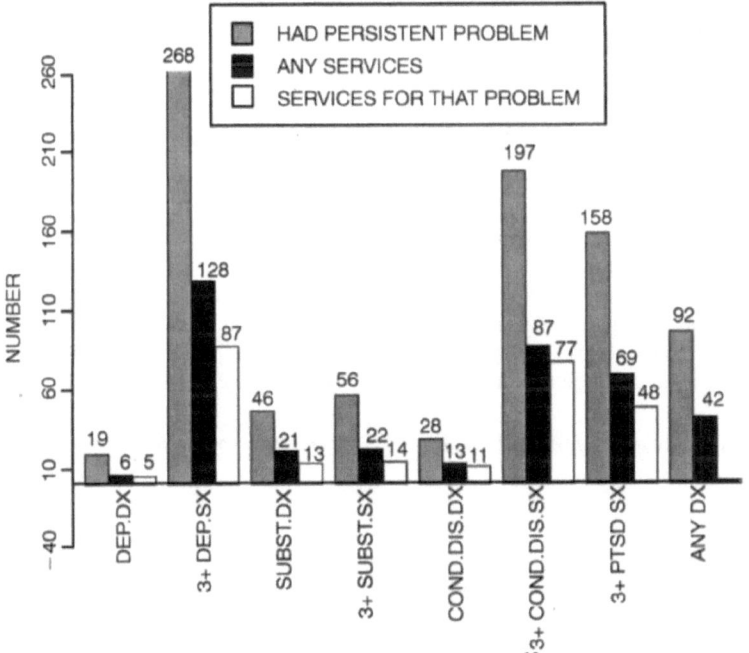

symptoms of depression than for youths who persistently met diagnostic criteria (48% to 32% for generic services and 33% to 26% for depression specific services). Similarly, service rates for youths with only persistent symptoms of substance abuse or conduct disorder did not differ from service rates for youths who persistently met diagnostic criteria for each problem (approximately 45% for generic services, with 27% for substance abuse specific help and 39% for conduct disorder specific help).

Which Providers Facilitate Youths' Access to Mental Health Services?

Obtaining mental health services requires that someone recognize the youth's problems and either provide services himself/herself or refer the youth to others for such help. Therefore, we used logistic regressions to examine the relationship between service use from 1994 to 1996 and contact with different categories of professionals in 1994, while controlling for age, gender, problem severity, and problem persistence. When controlling for sociodemographics and the presence and persistence of a mental health diagnosis, past contact with a social service provider was the only form of provider contact that significantly predicted later receipt of care for mental health problems between 1994 and 1996.

The odds ratios indicate that for each additional year of age, youths were less likely to receive services. Not surprisingly, youths meeting diagnostic criteria were almost twice as likely as other youths to receive services. Even after controlling for diagnosis, youths with persistent problems (diagnoses at both interviews) were twice as likely to receive services as youths whose problems were more transient. Youths in contact with the juvenile justice sector were only 1/2 as likely to receive services as other youths. Finally, of all the categories of helpers, only contact with a social service provider (even after controlling for diagnosis and persistence of problems) enhanced the likelihood that a youth would receive services over the course of the next two years (OR = 1.5). Contact with other categories of professionals made no significant difference in later service receipt (Table 1).

Who Provides the Mental Health Services that the Youths Receive?

Youths could receive services from only one provider, or from multiple providers. Thus some providers were alone in providing help, while others provided services at the same time as others were also doing so. We examined providers in five categories: MD/PhD mental health specialists, primary care MD, social service providers, teachers or coaches, and other helpers.

Over a two-year period, regardless of the severity of the youths' problems, more youths were helped by social service providers than by any other

TABLE 1. Logistic Regression Predicting Receipt of Services for Mental Health Problems Between 1994 and 1996, Controlling for Presence and Persistence of Diagnosis

Variable	Standardized Estimate	Wald Chi-Square	Odds Ratio
Intercept		1.7	
Age	−.10	4.8	.9*
Diagnosis in 1994 or 1996	.11	5.9	1.6**
Diagnosis in Both 1994 and 1996	.13	7.8	2.0**
From Juvenile Justice Sector	−.18	12.4	.5***
Saw a Social Service Provider in 1994	.10	4.7	1.5*

*p < .05, ** p < .01, *** p < .001
Model Chi-Square = 27.7, df = 5, p = .0001

category of provider (26.5% as compared to 3% to 15.3% served by other providers). This was true if youths received services from only one category of provider or from multiple categories. When served by only one provider, 12.6% of youths received mental health services from a social service provider as contrasted with less than 1% from an MD/PhD mental health specialist, 3% from a primary care MD, 4.7% from teachers, or 4.6% from others (see Figure 2). Similarly, when receiving help from multiple providers, 12.9% received help from a social service provider, as contrasted with 2.5% for an MD/PhD mental health specialist, 4.6% from a primary care MD, 7.4% from teachers, and 10.7% from others.

Which Providers Serve Youths with More Problems?

Figure 3 shows the distribution of professions helping youths who had persistent problems (met diagnostic criteria at two interviews). About 33% of those youths whose problems were persistent received services from a social service provider (12.6% from that provider alone, and 20.8% from multiple professionals). In contrast, only 4% received services from an MD/PhD level mental health specialist (1% alone, and 3.1% with other professionals); only

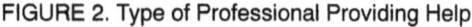

FIGURE 2. Type of Professional Providing Help

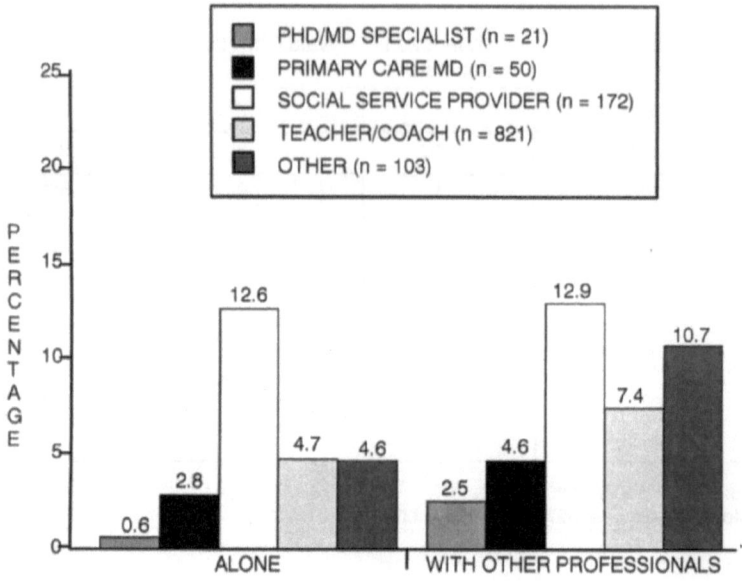

11.4% received help from a primary care MD (3.1% alone, and 8.3% with others); 17.7% received help from a teacher or coach (4.2% alone, and 13.5% with others); and 22% received help from others (4.2% alone, and 17.7% with other providers). Although not presented in this paper, a similar pattern of service provision was found for youths with only symptoms and for youths meeting diagnostic criteria at only one of the interviews.

It is noteworthy that, regardless of the severity of the youths' problems, social service professionals working alone served more youths than either MD/PhD mental health specialists or primary care physicians. One would expect that the MD/PhD specialists and other MD level providers would provide the bulk of services for youths meeting diagnostic criteria. These youths meet Medicaid and other insurance criteria for reimbursement, while other providers are often not eligible for reimbursement. However, for youths who met diagnostic criteria and for those who had the most persistent and severe problems, social service providers were still the only providers for almost as many youths as the reimbursable providers served with or without the presence of other helpers. The data clearly indicate the pivotal role social

FIGURE 3. If Had Persistent Diagnosis, Type of Professional Providing Help

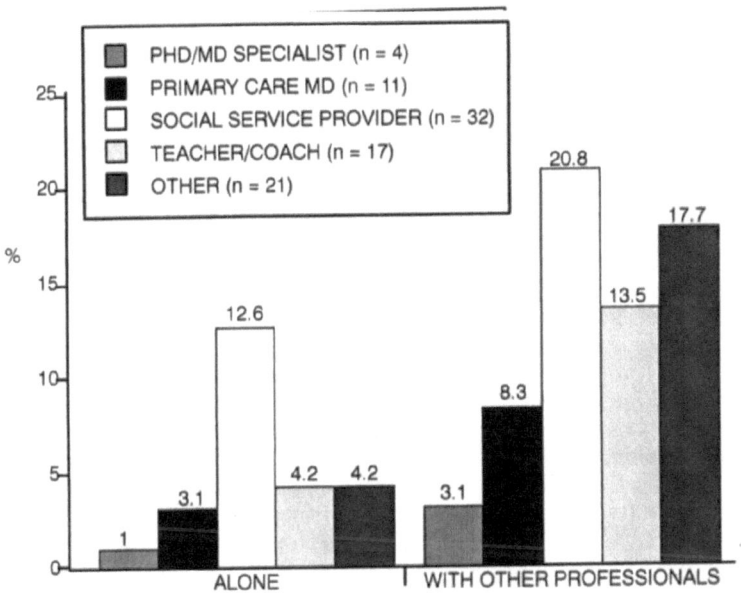

service providers play in both youths' pathways to mental health services and in their receipt of such services.

Does the Quality of Services Differ by Type of Profession?

Perception of help from services is an accepted, albeit not objective, method of measuring service quality (Seligman, 1996). In 1996, we asked youths how much they felt they had been helped by the different providers. When we asked all youths who received help, regardless of the severity or persistence of their problem, they reported being equivalently satisfied with services from a social service provider, teacher, other professional, or primary care MD. They were, however, significantly less satisfied with services provided by specialist MDs or PhDs. This pattern held for youths who met diagnostic criteria at only one of the two interviews. The patterns also held when we examined the responses of only those youths with persistent severe problems. They were less satisfied with services provided by MD/PhD level mental health specialists than they were with services provided by social service providers or others. The difference was not significant, in part because the sample size became too small. Therefore, regardless of their problems, youths' satisfaction with social service providers was always as high as their highest level of satisfaction with any service provider (see Table 2). One could respond that MD/PhD mental health specialists see youths who have more problems, and are thus likely to be more negative about the help they receive. However, our own data (Figure 3) show that those specialists do not see more troubled youths than do other providers.

DISCUSSION

Our findings support prior research that demonstrated a substantial gap between youths' need for mental health services and their receipt of services (Burns et al., 1995; Earls et al., 1989; Stiffman, Earls, Robins & Jung, 1988). The interviews showed that significant numbers of youths at each of the four sectors had mental health problems: both diagnoses and significant symptoms. However, only a limited percentage of those youths with mental health problems received services from their gateway sector.

The unique contribution of our study can be summarized in five points: (1) Contact with a social service provider, but not a physician or teacher or other professional, was associated with increased likelihood of receiving services regardless of the severity or persistence of a youth's problems; (2) Social service providers played a key role in both access to and provision of

TABLE 2. Mean Helpfulness of Services, by Type of Provider

Type of Provider:	All Youths Who Received Help		Youths with Diagnosis in Both 1994 and 1996	
	Mean	S.D.	Mean	S.D.
Specialist MD/PhD	1.9*	.81	1.5*	.58
Primary Care MD	2.3	.74	1.9	.78
Social Service Provider	2.4	.72	2.2	.80
Teacher/Coach	2.5	.60	2.4	.72
Other	2.4	.66	2.3	.75
Model Statistics	$R^2 = .03, p < .02$ df = 4,235		$R^2 = .06, p < .11$ df = 4,43	

*significantly different from other types of helpers

mental health services in all public sectors (education, juvenile justice, primary health, child welfare and mental health); (3) Social service providers provided help with behavioral or mental health problems to more youths than any other helping profession regardless of the severity of the youths' problems; (4) Social service providers provided the most services as the sole provider, and as one of many levels of providers; (5) Youths felt they had been helped at least as much by social service providers as by any other professionals.

Furthermore, because of the large percentage of service configurations in which multiple professionals helped a youth, our study illustrated the existence of a defacto treatment team, even if there is no contact or communication between the different helpers. This implies the need for enhanced communication and coordination so that the various providers can actually function together on behalf of the youth.

Though our findings suggest significant associations between need and service provision for a range of behavioral, emotional, and mental health problems, the reader should be aware of methodological issues that might affect the interpretation of our study. Since all the youth in our sample are from gateway sectors in only one Midwestern city, they or the gateway sector practices may not be representative of service users. We derive more confidence in the applicability of our results to St. Louis service users because the clinic records and anonymous tallies indicate that the youths in our sample are representative of teen clients from each public sector. Also, our data were collected through self-report via face-to-face interviews and respondents were asked for retrospective information over the previous 6 months. Depending on the question, responses may vary in their accuracy: for questions about illegal activities and violent behaviors, social desirability may have influenced responses; and for questions about past events, inaccurate memory and recall might have influenced responses. Finally, due to the great variety of youths' problems and services, the sample size was too small to examine the relationship between services and changes in specific symptoms or disorder.

This study focuses attention on several important issues for service delivery in multiple sectors of care. Managed care policies, which often limit mental health services to only the most severely impaired youths, and reimburse only MD/PhD level professionals, will inevitably direct more youths to social service sector providers (Proctor & Stiffman, 1998). Our study shows that social service providers are key to obtaining services. Further, they provide the bulk of services across the largest continuum of care, and appear to provide help of equal quality with other service providers. This information is critical for planning timely, appropriate, and cost effective interventions for a high risk underserved population, and for the education of social service professionals.

REFERENCES

Brandenburg, N. A., Friedman, R. M., & Silver, S. E. (1990). The epidemiology of childhood psychiatric disorders. *Journal of the American Academy of Child and Adolescent Psychiatry 29*(1), 76-83.

Burns, B. J., Costello, A. J., Angold, A., Tweed, D., Stangl, D., Farmer, E. M. Z., & Erkanli, A. (1995). Children's Mental Health Service Use Across Service Sectors. *Health Affairs, 14*, 147-159.

Burns, B. J., & Taube, C. A. (1989). Mental health services for adolescents: Background paper for the US Congress, Office of Technology Assessment.

Callicutt, J. W., & Lecca, P. J. (1983). The convergence of social work and mental health services. In J.W. Callicutt & P.J. Lecca (Eds.), *Social work and mental health* (pp. 3-10). New York: Free Press.

Cohen, P., Kasen, S., Brook, J. S., & Struening, E. L. (1991). Diagnostic predictors of treatment patterns in a cohort of adolescents. *Journal of the American Academy of Child and Adolescent Psychiatry 30*(6), 989-993.

Cohen, P., Velez, N., Kohn, M., Schwab-Stone, M., & Johnson, J. (1987). Child psychiatric diagnosis by computer algorithm: Theoretical issues and empirical tests. *Journal of the American Academy of Child and Adolescent Psychiatry 26*, 631-638.

Consumer Reports. (1995) Mental Health: Does Therapy Help? November, 734-739.

Costello, E. J. (1989). Developments in child psychiatric epidemiology. *Journal of the American Academy of Child and Adolescent Psychiatry 28*, 836-841.

Costello, E. J., Angold, A., Burns, B. J., Farmer, E. M. Z., Stangl, D. K., Erkanli, A., & Messerm, S. C. (1995). *Great Smoky Mountains study: 1. Use of services for mental health care.* NIMH Mental Health Services Research Conference.

Costello, E.J., Burns, B.J., Costello, A.J., Edelbrock, C., Dulcan, M., & Brent, D. (1988). Service utilization and psychiatric diagnosis in pediatric primary care: The role of the gatekeeper. *Pediatrics, 82*(3/2), 435-441.

Earls, F., Robins, L. N., Stiffman, A. R., & Powell, J. (1989). Comprehensive health care for high risk adolescents: An evaluation study. *American Journal of Public Health, 79*, 999-1105.

Garland, A. F. (1995). *Teachers' identification of adolescents' need for mental health services.* NIMH Mental Health Services Research Conference.

Harold, N. B., & Harold, R. D. (1993). School-based clinics: A response to the physical and mental health needs of adolescents. *Health and Social Work, 18*, 65-74.

Horwitz, S. M., Hoagwood, K., Stiffman, A. R., Summerfelt, T., Weisz, J. R., Costello, E. J., Rost, R., Bean, D. L., Cottler, L., Leaf, P. J., Roper, M., & Norquist, G. (In review). Measuring Youths' Use of Mental Health Services: Reliability of the SACA–The Services Assessment for Children and Adolescents.

Horwitz, S.M., Leaf, P.J., Leventhal, J.M., Borsyth, B., & Speechley, K.N. (1992). Identification and management of psychosocial and developmental problems in community-based, primary care pediatric practices. *Pediatrics, 89*(3), 480-485.

Landsverk, J. (In press). Foster care and pathways to mental health services. P. Curtis & G. Dale (Eds.), *The foster care crisis: Translating research into practice and policy.* Lincoln, NE: University of Nebraska Press.

Lourie, I. (1987). New approaches in mental health services for adolescents. *The Clinical Psychologist, 40*(4), 85-87.

Lourie, I. S., & Katz-Leavy, J. (1991). New directions for mental health services for families and children. *Families in Society: The Journal of Contemporary Human Services,* May, 277-285.

Marino, S., Gallo, J.J., Ford, D.E., & Anthony, J.C. (1995). Filters on the pathway to mental health care, I. Incident mental disorders. *Psychological Medicine, 25,* 1135-1148.

Offord, D. R., Boyle, M. H., Flemin, J. E., Blum, H. M., & Rae-Grant, N. I. (1989). Ontario child health study: Summary of selected results. *Canadian Journal of Psychiatry, 34,* 483-491.

Pescosolido, B.A. (1992). Beyond rational choice: The social dynamics of how people seek help. *American Journal of Sociology, 97* (4), 1096-1138.

Proctor, E. P., & Stiffman, A. R. (In press). Mental Health Treatment and Service Research: Background. In Williams, J. B. W. & Ell, K. (Eds.) *Recent Advances in Mental Health Research: Implications for Social Work Practice.* NASW Press.

Saunders, S. M., Resnick, M.D., Hoberman, H. M., & Blum, R. W. (1994). Formal help-seeking behavior of adolescents identifying themselves as having mental health problems. *Journal of the American Academy of Child and Adolescent Psychiatry, 33,* 718-728.

Schaffer, D., Schwab-Stone, M., Fisher, P., & Cohen, P. et al. (1993). The Diagnostic Interview Schedule for Children-Revised Version (DISC-R): I. Preparation, field testing, interrater reliability, and acceptability. *Journal of the American Academy of Child and Adolescent Psychiatry, 32,* 643-650.

Seligman, M.E.P. (1996). A Creditable Beginning. *American Psychologist, 51,* 1086-1087.

StataCorp (1997). Stata Statistical Software: Release 5.0. College Station, TX: Stata Corporation.

Stiffman, A. R., Chen, Y. W., Elze, D., Doré, P., & Cheng, L. C. (1997). Adolescents' and providers' perspectives on the need for and use of mental health services. *Journal of Adolescent Health, 21* (5), 335-342.

Stiffman, A.R., & Cunningham, R. (1990). The epidemiology of child and adolescent mental health disorders, in Gibbs J.T. (ed.). *Child and Adolescent Mental Health: Challenges for Social Work Education and Practice.* (pp. 9-32) NASW Press: Berkeley CA, University of California.

Stiffman, A. R., Earls, F., Robins, L.N., & Jung, K. (1988). Problems and help-seeking in high-risk adolescent patients of health clinics. *Journal of Adolescent Health Care, 9,* 305-309.

Stiffman, A. R., Horwitz, S. M., Hoagwood, K., Compton, W., Cottler, L., Bean, D. L., Narrow, W. & Weisz, J. R. (In review). Adult and child reports of mental health services in the Service Assessment for Children and Adolescents (SACA).

Taube, P. S., & Barrett, S. A. (1983). Mental health: United States 1983. *DHHS Publication No. ADM 83-1275.* Washington, DC: U.S. Government Printing Office.

Depression Treatment and Cost Offset for Rural Community Residents with Depression

Mingliang Zhang
Kathryn M. Rost
John C. Fortney

SUMMARY. This study examined the relationship between costs of treating physical problems and costs of treating depression, for 322 rural residents with depression. Multiple regressions were used to control for sociodemographics, depression severity, and physical and mental health comorbidities at baseline. The results indicated a $1.42 (n = 322) reduction in the costs of treating physical problems for a $1.00

Mingliang Zhang is affiliated with the Outcomes Research Department at Merck & Co., Inc. Kathryn M. Rost is Research Health Scientist and Associate Professor, Centers for Mental Healthcare Research, Department of Psychiatry, University of Arkansas for Medical Sciences, Little Rock, AR. John C. Fortney is Research Health Scientist and Assistant Professor, Veterans Administration Health Services Research & Development Field Program, Veterans Administration Medical Center, Little Rock, AR.

Address correspondence to: Mingliang Zhang, Outcomes Research Department, Merck & Co., Inc., P.O. Box 100, WS1B-70, One Merck Drive, Whitehouse Station, NJ 08889.

This research is supported by grants from the National Institute of Mental Health (MH48197, MH55297, MH54444, and MH49116) and Veterans Affairs Administration (HFP90-019). The authors thank Gregory Simon, MD, for his comments on an earlier draft of the paper. Some of the results were presented at the NIMH 11th International Conference on Mental Health Problems in the General Health Care Sector.

[Haworth co-indexing entry note]: "Depression Treatment and Cost Offset for Rural Community Residents with Depression." Zhang, Mingliang, Kathryn M. Rost, and John C. Fortney. Co-published simultaneously in *Journal of Social Service Research* (The Haworth Press, Inc.) Vol. 25, No. 3, 1999, pp. 99-110; and: *Mental Health Services and Sectors of Care* (ed: Enola K. Proctor, Nancy Morrow-Howell, and Arlene Stiffman) The Haworth Press, Inc., 1999, pp. 99-110. Single or multiple copies of this article are available for a fee from The Haworth Document Delivery Service [1-800-342-9678, 9:00 a.m. - 5:00 p.m. (EST). E-mail address: getinfo@haworthpressinc.com].

increase in the costs of treating depression. The reduction was $2.61 (p < 0.05) among those receiving depression treatment (n = 125). These findings suggest a net savings from depression treatment, in addition to other benefits such as improved symptoms and functioning and increased productivity. *[Article copies available for a fee from The Haworth Document Delivery Service: 1-800-342-9678. E-mail address: getinfo@haworth pressinc.com]*

KEYWORDS. Cost offset, depression, rural

INTRODUCTION

Depression is a common mental disorder in the general U.S. population. The most recent estimate from the National Comorbidity Survey (Kessler et al., 1994) indicates that the 1-year prevalence of unipolar major depression and dysthymia among community residents aged 15 to 54 years is 10.3%, about 27 million Americans today. An additional 11% of community residents who do not meet the strict criteria for either depressive disorder are estimated to have substantial depressive symptoms (Depression Guideline Panel, 1993). Recent estimates of costs of treatment for depressive disorders range between $12.4 billion (Greenberg et al., 1993) and $19.2 billion (Rice and Miller, 1993) per year in 1990 dollars. Even the most carefully derived estimates do not include the treatment costs for primary care services when depression is treated, but not coded (Rost et al., 1994).

It has been shown in a large staff-model HMO that patients with a diagnosis of depression have greater chronic physical illness than patients without the diagnosis of depression (Unutzer et al., 1997). This possibility of exacerbated physical problems associated with depression supports a hypothesis that treating depression may reduce the need for treating physical problems and, therefore, the costs of treating depression may be offset by the reduced costs of treating physical problems. Health services researchers have long been interested in this cost offset effect in depression treatment in particular and in mental health services in general. Numerous studies, particularly in alcohol research, have investigated the cost offset phenomenon (Jones and Vischi, 1979; Holder and Blose, 1986; Mumford et al., 1984; Booth et al., 1997). The theory of cost offset arises from research substantiating that undiagnosed individuals with mental and substance abuse disorders use large quantities of general medical care, frequently receiving health services unrelated to their underlying mental health or substance abuse disorder (Jones and Vischi, 1979; Holder, 1987). However, after receiving appropriate mental health or substance abuse services, use of services for physical problems may be reduced, presumably because of reductions in symptomatology and medical complications. It is important that society's decision to allocate scarce resources should be based on cost-effectiveness, the outcomes achieved by the services. However, because of today's spiraling health care costs and thus the need for cost containment, the existence of a cost offset effect in addition to improved outcomes offers a uniquely strong argument for financing mental health services.

This paper investigates whether there is a cost offset effect in depression treatment from a rural community sample of individuals with major depression, dysthymia, and substantial depressive symptoms. Although previous cost offset studies in alcohol research literature have rendered mixed results (Holder, 1987; Booth et al., 1997), no study has been published in individuals with depression to investigate whether cost offset exists in this population. We focus our analyses in rural community residents because in rural areas health services, particularly mental health services, are less available because of fewer health care providers; less accessible because of geographical distances and the lack of public transportation (Cuffel, 1994); less acceptable culturally because of greater stigma associated with seeking mental health services (Rost et al., 1993); and less affordable because rural residents are more likely to be poor (Rowland and Lyons, 1989). These barriers to accessing mental health services in rural areas are likely to result in substituting physical health services for their mental health problems. These physical health services, particularly in hospital settings, result in high health care costs, yet without improvement in patients' mental health outcomes. Therefore, rural patients with depression afford the greatest potential for a cost offset effect.

METHODS

Data Collection

Using a stratified sampling design to oversample rural subjects, 11,078 individuals from 15,721 households in Arkansas with listed or unlisted telephone numbers were selected to complete an 8-item screener (Burnam et al., 1988) for current depression. Of these, 998 (9%) screened positive for depressive disorder or substantial depressive symptoms. The screener exhibited 89% sensitivity and 95% specificity values in community samples, compared to the Diagnostic Interview Schedule (DIS) (Robins et al., 1989) diagnosis of major depression or dysthymia in the past month (Burnam et al., 1988).

Subjects who screened positive were excluded from the study if they:

(1) exhibited acute suicidal ideation (n = 14), (2) reported that depressed mood began following a bereavement (n = 288), (3) were subsequently diagnosed with lifetime mania (n = 54), or (4) denied all depressive symptoms in the extended baseline interview (n = 8). Of the 634 individuals eligible for the study, 470 (74%) agreed to participate in the longitudinal study. The data were collected in 3 stages: an extended baseline interview, and 6-month and 12-month follow-up interviews. The extended baseline interview was conducted at subjects' homes and the follow-up interviews were done by telephone. The depression section of the DIS (Robins et al., 1989) was used to diagnose lifetime and current major depression and dysthymia. Subjects who did not meet criteria for a depressive disorder were categorized as having substantial symptoms of depression, a group with levels of functional impairment comparable to those of the group meeting criteria (Wells et al., 1989).

To collect utilization/charge information, subjects were asked to provide consent for release of information from all providers (physicians, psychologists, social workers, counselors, nurse practitioners, physician assistants, chiropractors, hospitals, emergency rooms, clinics, and pharmacies) and third party payers of health care during the previous 6 months at the 6- and 12-month interviews. At the end of the 12-month interview, both health care providers and third-party payers were contacted to obtain all essential medical records and billing/reimbursement records. These records were also used to identify additional health care providers that were not identified by subjects at the 6-month and 12-month interviews. Medical and billing records from these additional providers were then obtained. This process, though labor intensive, has been used in several successful projects (Smith et al., 1986; Kashner et al., 1992) to collect utilization and expenditure data in a community population.

We examined differences between participants and nonparticipants (eligible individuals who refused to participate in the longitudinal study) of the longitudinal study. Of all sociodemographic and clinical variables examined, only age was found to differ significantly (p < 0.01) between the participant and nonparticipant groups. Gender, race, marital status, insurance coverage, baseline severity, physical and psychiatric comorbidities, previous health care utilization (self-report at baseline), and lost work days were not found to differ significantly. Because participants and nonparticipants did not differ in utilization, severity and comorbidity, the effect of non-response bias in estimating costs of treatment is expected to be minimal. To increase the representativeness of the sample and to adjust for the stratified sample design, we weighted the sample by age, gender, education, and region so that our sample more closely resembled the rural depressed adults we identified as eligible for the study.

The follow-up rate was 97.8% at 6 months (excluding 5 subjects who died before the 6-month follow-up) and 98.5% at 12 months (excluding 2 subjects who died between the 6- and 12-month interviews). Of the 470 subjects participating in the study, 446 (94.9%) completed both the 6-month and 12-month follow-up interviews. We were not able to obtain complete medical and insurance records for 11 of these subjects and they were excluded. Of the final sample of 435 subjects with complete utilization/expenditure information, 322 were rural residents. In this paper, we focused our analyses on these 322 rural subjects. However, we performed a sensitivity analysis by expanding the sample to include both the rural and urban subjects (n = 435).

Determination of Costs of Treatment

In order to calculate the costs of treatment for depression and for physical problems as accurately as possible, a reliable methodology was developed to abstract charge data from medical and billing/reimbursement records. The first author of this paper conducted a 1-week training session for abstractors using a detailed protocol he developed for abstracting utilization/charge data from these records. During the training session, the abstractors and the first author compared the results of abstracting they completed independently on 10 selected subjects, analyzed reasons for discrepant coding decisions, established new rules as needed, and incorporated all rules into the final written protocol. Following this final protocol, the abstracted data by each abstractor were compared to that by the first author to determine the percentage of concordance in abstraction between the two. This percentage is used to measure the inter-rater reliability between the abstractor and the first author. Then, the mean inter-rater reliability among all the abstractors independently rating 10 subjects was determined to be 90.8% initially and 89.9% after one-third of the records had been abstracted.

When medical and insurance records indicated depression as the sole diagnosis, all charges associated with the hospitalization/visit were attributed to depression treatment except for procedures unrelated to depression (e.g., chest x-rays, Pap smears, allergy injections), which were attributed to treatment for physical problems. When depression treatment was provided during hospitalizations wherein patients primarily received care for physical problems, 2 psychiatrists independently reviewed the medical and billing records to allocate the proportion of charges relevant to depression and to physical problems. When the 2 psychiatrists disagreed about the amount of charges attributable to the treatment of depression, we deferred to the higher estimate. When depression treatment was provided during outpatient visits during which the patient received care for physical problems, we allocated 50% of the charges for the visit to depression treatment. The remainder of the charges was allocated to care for physical problems. A similar procedure was used to allocate charges when the visit addressed multiple psychiatric problems including depression. All health care costs were converted into 1994 4th-quarter values using the medical component of the consumer price index (CPI) (U.S. Department of Commerce, 1994).

Definitions of Other Major Variables

Rurality–a subject is defined as living in a rural area if his/her county of residence is not in a metropolitan statistical area (MSA).

Physical comorbidity–measured by the number of 11 chronic physical conditions reported by a subject at baseline. They included arthritis, asthma, cancer, diabetes, epilepsy, heart disease, chronic lung disease, gastrointestinal disorders, hypertension, renal failure, and stroke.

Psychiatric comorbidity–identified at baseline by the Quick Diagnostic Interview Schedule (QDIS) (Marcus et al., 1991), included lifetime and 1-year anxiety, panic, obsessive/compulsive disorder, alcohol dependence or abuse, drug dependence or abuse, schizophrenia/schizophreniform, and posttraumatic stress disorders.

Depression severity–measured by the acuity of DSM-III-R depressive symptoms, standardized to a 0-10 scale.

Sociodemographic variables–included age, gender, education, marital status, minority status, employment status, and income. Income is expressed as the ratio of family income to the poverty level of the corresponding family size for each subject.

Analytical Model

In order to examine the relationship between the costs of treatment for physical health and the costs of treatment for depression, we specified a multiple regression model where cost of treatment for physical problems for the year (baseline to 12-month follow-up) was the dependent variable and cost of depression treatment for the year was the explanatory variable, controlling for sociodemographics, baseline physical and psychiatric comorbidities, and baseline depression severity. We examined the effect on expected costs of treatment for physical problems for an additional dollar increase in the costs for treatment of depression, or the marginal cost offset effect. This model was applied initially to all subjects in rural areas (n = 322) and subsequently to rural subjects who received depression treatment (n = 125). Because of the skewness of the cost distribution, a logarithm transformation was applied to the costs of physical health and the expected costs of physical health were retransformed from the estimations using a non-parametric method (Duan, 1983).

RESULTS

Overall, 59.2% of the subjects were female, 20.1% were minorities (predominantly African-American), and 64.1% were married. The average age was 47.2 years (range 18-86). The average income-to-poverty ratio was 2.4 (range 0.2-8.7). The subjects had an average of 2.7 (range 0-9) physical comorbidities and 1.1 (0-8) psychiatric comorbidities. The average standardized DIS score for depression severity at baseline was 5.0 (0-10 scale). The average annual expenditures were $4,775.89 (range $0-$59,597.29) for physical problems and $195.11 (range $0-$8,153.96) for depression. Among those receiving any depression treatment (N = 125), the average annual expenditures were $7,328.89 (range $0-$59,597.29) for physical problems and $473.72 (range $0-$8,153.96) for depression.

The regression results are presented in Table 1. After re-transformation (not shown in the table), the coefficient on depression treatment costs from the first regression (n = 322), calculated as the marginal effect at the mean, is − 1.42 controlling for depression severity, physical and psychiatric comorbidities, and sociodemographics. This result implies that there is a $1.42 decrease in the costs of treatment for physical problems for an additional $1.00 increase in the costs of any treatment for depression. In other words, there is

TABLE 1. Regression Results[†]

Variables	Regression 1	Regression 2
Intercept	1.55	1.14**
Age (age/10)	0.47**	0.35
Gender (female = 1)	0.75*	0.26
Education (0-9 scale)	− 0.11	0.05
Marital status (married = 1)	− 0.39	0.49
Income-to-poverty ratio	0.31**	− 0.02
Employment (employed = 1)	− 0.32	− 0.18
Race (white = 1)	0.08	− 0.75
Number of physical comorbidities	0.38**	0.24*
Number of psychiatric comorbidities	0.23*	0.23
Depression severity (0-10 scale)	0.17**	0.06
Depression treatment costs ($1,000)	− 0.29	− 0.47*
N	322	125
R^2	0.26	0.20

†The dependent variable is the logarithm of the costs for treating physical health problems. Regression 1 is for all rural subjects (n = 322) and regression 2 is for those rural subjects who received depression treatment (n = 125).
*$p < 0.05$; **$p < 0.01$.

a net return of 42% for treating depression in the rural community. Among the rural subjects who received depression treatment (the second regression, n = 125), there is an overall $2.61 (p < 0.05) decrease in costs of treating physical health problems associated with $1.00 increase in costs of depression treatment, or a 161% net return.

Sensitivity Analyses

In determining costs of outpatient visits where the purpose was for depression and other problems, we arbitrarily assumed 50% of costs were for depression. We performed sensitivity analyses by assuming this allocation to be 0% and 100%, respectively. The overall cost offset results for rural subjects remained to be true. However, in another sensitivity analysis where we expanded the sample to also include the urban subjects (for a total of 435 subjects), there was only a $0.24 decrease (not statistically significant) in the cost for treating physical problems for every $1.00 increase in depression treatment.

DISCUSSION

An additional $1.00 increase in the costs of depression treatment in rural areas is associated with a substantial cost offset effect on the cost of treating physical problems. Although the result for the whole sample (n = 322) is not statistically significant (p = 0.14), we believe it is worth reporting because of its magnitude. Cost distributions are usually highly skewed and very large samples are needed to detect cost differences in the conventional statistical levels, unless the difference is extremely large such as the case in our subsample of the 125 treated subjects (i.e., a 161% net return on cost of depression treatment).

However, treatment costs are only a small portion of the total cost of depression to society. The consensus reached by a national panel points out that depression is seriously undertreated, resulting in large costs to society (Hirschfeld et al., 1997). Estimates of costs due to mortality and morbidity (disability and lost productivity) (Broadhead et al., 1990; Korff et al., 1992; Ormel et al., 1993; Klerman and Weissman, 1992; Johnson et al., 1992; Mintz et al., 1992) range from $11.2 billion (Rice and Miller, 1993) to $31.3 billion (Greenberg et al., 1993) in 1990 dollars, representing 41.6% to 72.0% of the total costs of depression to society. Yet these estimates of indirect costs are conservative because they do not include costs to family caregivers (Franks, 1990; Stommel et al., 1994), lost leisure time (Leigh and Fries, 1992), or the pain and suffering endured by depressed individuals and their families (Bartel and Taubman, 1986).

A cost offset effect associated with depression treatment is an added benefit of treatment and it (or lack of) should not be used as the sole basis of a decision to finance treatment for depression in particular, and mental health services in general. Such a decision should be based on the outcomes achieved by the services, i.e., cost-effectiveness. These outcomes include changes in the severity of depressive symptoms, improved participation in the labor market, fewer missed work days and unproductive days, reduced pain and suffering, and improved quality of life for the patients and their family. The costs of treatment should be measured against the overall outcomes (including potential cost offset) the treatment achieves in making policy decisions as to whether and how depression treatment should be financed.

Nevertheless, our findings indicate that cost offset of depression treatment exists in rural populations, but not in urban populations. This probably reflects the fact that there are fewer providers, especially mental health providers, in rural areas than in urban areas. As a result, medical services, particularly inpatient services, are substituted in rural areas. Our analyses in another study using this same database indicate that rural subjects use significantly fewer mental health specialty care visits for depression but they are 3.05 times more likely to be hospitalized for physical problems during a year (Rost et al., 1997). Our findings support the need of policies designed to promote awareness, detection, and treatment of depression in rural areas, where providers, particularly mental health providers, are less available than in urban areas.

Our analyses only indicate an association, not a causal relationship, between treatment for depression and treatment for physical problems. It is possible that chronic physical illnesses may be exacerbated by depression and therefore treating depression may reduce the need and intensity for treating physical problems. It is also possible, on the other hand, that chronic physical illnesses increase the risk of depression. Therefore, the presence of physical problems may lead to increased costs for treating depression. Furthermore, depression might increase reporting of somatic distress and increase the likelihood that physical illnesses are reported and treated.

While our conclusions are strengthened by the study's prospective design with a community-based sample, high follow-up rates, and the extensive procedure we employed to determine utilization, we also acknowledge limitations to the generalizability of our findings. First, because we recruited our cohort using a telephone survey, we eliminated approximately 11% of the state's residents who were without a household telephone. Second, because few subjects were covered by capitated insurance plans, we do not know whether these findings generalize to regions where capitation dominates. Third, costs have a highly skewed distribution and large samples are needed to detect a statistically significant difference. Our sample size is relatively small. Future studies may be designed to address these issues.

REFERENCES

Bartel, A. and P. Taubman, 1986, Some economic and demographic consequences of mental illness. *Journal of Labor Economics 4*(2), 243-256.

Booth, B.M., F.C. Blow, C.A.L. Cook, J.Y. Bunn, and J.C. Fortney, 1996, Relationship between inpatient alcoholism treatment and longitudinal changes in health care utilization. *Journal of Studies on Alcohol 58*(6), 625-637.

Broadhead, W.E., D.G. Blazer, L.K. George, and C.K. Tse, 1990, Depression, disability days, and days lost from work in a prospective epidemiologic survey. *Journal of the American Medical Association 264*(19), 2524-2528.

Burnam, M.A., K.B. Wells, B. Leake, and J. Landsverk, 1988, Development of a brief screening instrument for detecting depressive disorders. *Medical Care 26* (8), 775-789.

Cuffel, B.J. 1994, Violent and destructive behavior among the severely mentally ill in rural areas: Evidence from Arkansas's community mental health system. *Community Mental Health Journal 30*(5), 495-504.

Depression Guideline Panel, 1993, Depression in primary care: Volume 1. Detection and diagnosis. Clinical practice guideline, Number 5. (AHCPR Publication No. 93-0550), (US Department of Health and Human Services, Public Health Service, Agency for Health Care Policy and Research).

Duan, N. 1983, Smearing estimate: A nonparametric retransformation method. *Journal of the American Statistical Association 78*(383), 605-610.

Franks, D.D. 1990, Economic contribution of families caring for persons with severe and persistent mental illness. *Administration and Policy in Mental Health 18*(1), 9-18.

Greenberg, P.E., L.E. Stiglin, S.N. Finkelstein, and E.R. Berndt, 1993, The economic burden of depression in 1990. *Journal of Clinical Psychiatry 54*, 405-418.

Hirschfeld, R., M.B. Keller, S. Panico, B.S. Arons, D. Barlow, F. Davidoff, J. Endicott, J. Froom, M. Goldstein, J.M. Gorman, D. Guthrie, R.G. Marek, T.A. Maurer, R. Meyer, K. Phillips, J. Ross, T.L. Schwenk, S.S. Sharfstein, M.E. Thase, and R.J. Wyatt, 1997, The National Depressive and Manic-Depressive Association consensus statement on the undertreatment of depression. *Journal of the American Medical Association 277*, 333-340.

Holder, H.D. 1987, Alcoholism treatment and potential health care cost saving. *Medical Care 25* (1), 52-71.

Holder, H.D. and J.O. Blose, 1986, Alcoholism treatment and total health care utilization costs: A four-year longitudinal analysis of federal employees. *Journal of the American Medical Association 256* (11), 1456-1460.

Johnson, J., M.M. Weissman, and G.L. Klerman, 1992, Service utilization and social morbidity associated with depressive symptoms in the community. *Journal of the American Medical Association 267*(11), 1478-1483.

Jones, K.R. and T.R. Vischi, 1979, Impact of alcohol, drug abuse and mental health treatment on medical care utilization: A review of the research literature. *Medical Care 17*(S), 1-82.

Kashner, T.M., K. Rost, G.R. Smith, Jr., and S. Lewis, 1992, An analysis of panel data: The impact of a psychiatric consultation letter on the expenditures and outcomes of care for patients with somatization disorder. *Medical Care 30*(9), 811-821.

Kessler, R.C., K.A. McGonagle, S. Zhao, C.B. Nelson, M. Hughes, S. Eshleman, H.U. Wittchen, and K.S. Kendler, 1994, Lifetime and 12-month prevalence of DSM-III-R psychiatric disorders in the United States: Results from the National Comorbidity Survey. *Archives of General Psychiatry 51*(1), 8-19.

Klerman, G.L. and M.M. Weissman, 1992, The course, morbidity, and costs of depression. *Archives of General Psychiatry 49*, 831-834.

Korff, M.V., J. Ormel, W. Katon, and E.H.B. Lin, 1992, Disability and depression among high utilizers of health care: A longitudinal analysis. *Archives of General Psychiatry 49*, 91-100.

Leigh, J.P. and J.F. Fries, 1992, Health habits, health care use and costs in a sample of retirees. *Inquiry 29*, 44-54.

Marcus, S., L.N. Robins, and K. Bucholz, 1991, Quick Diagnostic Interview Schedule III-R: Version 1.0. (Washington University School of Medicine, St. Louis).

Mintz, J., L.I. Mintz, M.J. Arruda, and S.S. Hwang, 1992, Treatments of depression and the functional capacity to work. *Archives of General Psychiatry 49*, 761-768.

Mumford, E., H.J. Schlesinger, G.V. Glass, C. Patrick, and T. Cuerdon, 1984, A new look at evidence about reduced costs of medical utilization following mental health treatment. *American Journal of Psychiatry 141*, 1145-1158.

Ormel, J., M. Von Korff, W. van den Brink, W. Katon, E. Brilman, and T. Oldehinkel, 1993, Depression, anxiety, and social disability show synchrony of change in primary care patients. *American Journal of Public Health 83*, 285-390.

Rice, D.P. and L.S. Miller, 1993, The economic burden of affective disorders. *Advances in Health Economics and Health Services Research 14*, 21-37.

Robins, L., J. Helzer, L. Cottler, and E. Goldring, 1989, NIMH Diagnostic Interview Schedule, Version III Revised (DIS-III-R). [Unpublished].

Rost, K.M., G.R. Smith, B. Guise, and D. Matthews, 1994, The deliberate misdiagnosis of major depression in primary care. *Archives of Family Medicine 3*, 333-337.

Rost, K., M. Zhang, J.C. Fortney, J.L. Smith, and G.R. Smith, 1998, Rural-urban differences in depression treatment and suicidality. *Med Care* Vol. 36 (7), 1098-1107.

Rost, K.M., G.R. Smith, and J.L. Taylor, 1993, Rural-urban differences in stigma and the use of care for depressive disorders. *Journal of Rural Health 9*(1), 57-62.

Rowland, D. and B. Lyons, 1989, Triple jeopardy: Rural, poor, and uninsured. *Health Services Research 23*(6), 975-1004.

Smith, G.R., Jr., R.A. Monson, and D.C. Ray, 1986, Psychiatric consultation in somatization disorder: A randomized, controlled study. *New England Journal of Medicine 314*, 1407-1413.

Stommel, M., C.E. Collins, and B.A. Given, 1994, The costs of family contributions to the care of persons with dementia. *Gerontologist 34*(2), 199-205.

U.S. Department of Commerce, 1994, Statistical Abstract of the United States 1994, 114th ed.

Unutzer, J., D.L. Patrick, G. Simon, D. Grembowski, E. Walker, C. Rutter, and W. Katon, 1997, Depressive symptoms and the cost of health services in HMO patients aged 65 years and older–A 4-year prospective study. *Journal of the American Medical Association 277* (20), 1618-1623.

Wells, K.B., A. Stewart, R.D. Hays, M.A. Burnam, W. Rogers, M. Daniels, S. Berry, S. Greenfield, and J. Ware, 1989, The functioning and well-being of depressed patients: Results from the Medical Outcomes Study. *Journal of the American Medical Association 262*, 914-919.

Index

Adoption and Child Welfare
    Assistance Act, 7
African Americans
    emergency shelter facility and, 13
    See also Minority factors
Age factors
    children's service systems
        reactivity and, 42,45,
        47,51,54
    in multiple service systems, 13
Alcohol abuse
    measures of, 87
    rural community residents and,
        100,101,104
    treatment and, 88
Antisocial behavior, as externalized
    behavior, 43
Asian/Pacific Islander youth
    Emergency shelter facilities and, 13
    See also Minority factors
Assessment
    in child welfare system, 6,7
    in emergency shelter facilities, 8,17

Badger, Lee W., 21
Berbaum, Michael, 21

Carney, Patricia A., 21
CBCL. *See* Child Behavior Checklist
Center for the Study of Social Policy,
    42
Child Behavior Checklist (CBCL),
    47,48
Child welfare system
    abused children and, 6
    antisocial behavior and, 42

    cost-effective interventions and, 8
    early problem identification and, 7
    emotionally disturbed children and,
        42,61-64
    functioning of youth and, 6
    as gateway for mental health
        services, 6,7,8,16,84
    interagency collaboration and,
        61-63
    kinship placement and, 7
    multiple placements and, 2,44,
        48-49,50
    neglected children and, 42
    network analysis and, 62
    out-of-home placement and,
        2,6,7,63
    screening assessments and, 6,7
    See also Children's service systems
Children
    aggression and, 43
    antisocial behavior and, 43
    anxiety and, 43
    depression and, 43
    disobedience and, 43
    stealing and, 43
    See also Children's service
        systems; Child welfare
        system
The Children's Initiative in North
    Carolina, 64
Children's service systems
    externalizing behavior problems
        and, 43-48,51,53,54,55,56,57
    internalizing mental health
        problems and, 43-48,51,53,
        54,55,56,57
    minority vs. non-minority factors
        and, 1,47,49,50,51-53,55,57
    network analysis and, 62

   111

placement ejections and, 44,45,50
psychosocial problems and, 45,56
reactivity in, 41
    age factors and,
        42,45,47,50,51,54
    gender factors and,
        42,45,47,50,51,54
    indicators of, 44,48-49
    minority factors,
        1,47,49,50,51-53,55,57
    responsiveness relative to, 45
residential placements and,
    44,50,56
responsiveness in, 41,43-44
    alcohol abuse treatment and, 48
    gender factors and,
        42,45,47,50,51,54
    indicators of, 48
    minority factors,
        1,47,49,50,51-53,55,57
    reactivity relative to, 45
    substance abuse treatment and,
        48
service workers, training of, 56
state custody focus and,
    41-57,61-64
study discussion, 55-57
study hypotheses, 45-47
study methodology, 47-48
    data analysis and, 50-51
    ordinal variables and, 49-50
    system reactivity indicators,
        48-49
    system responsiveness
        indicators, 48
study results
    alternate structural models, 55
    sample characteristics, 51
    sample comparability, 51
    test of hypothesized model,
        53-55
    tests of measurement model,
        51-53
See also Child welfare system
Criminal justice system, prior
        involvement and, 2,5,6,12

Depression
    diagnosis of by primary care
        physician, 22
    gender factors and, 23
    internalized behavior and, 43
    pharmacological options and,
        23,31,32,33,35
    recognition by primary care
        physician, 22,34,35,36
    rural community residents and,
        99-107
        cost offsets and, 101
        cultural stigma and, 101
        mental health services,
            accessibility and, 101
        physical illness comorbidity
            and, 100,101,102
        poverty and, 101
        primary care services and, 100
        resource allocation, 101
        treatment costs and, 100
    See also Depression treatment
Depression treatment
    gender factors and, 23
    general medical care and, 100
    pharmacological options and,
        31,32,33
    physical illness comorbidity and,
        100,101,102
    psychosocial presentations and,
        24,26,27,28,29,30,31,32,34
    rural community cost offsets and,
        99-107
        study discussion and, 106-108
        study methods and, analytical
            model and, 104
        study methods and, 101-104
        study methods and, data
            collection and, 101-103
        study methods and, definitions
            used in, 104
        study methods and, treatment
            cost factors and, 103-104
        study results and, 105-106
    somatic symptoms and, 26,27,28,
        29,30,32,34

study discussion, 106-107
study introduction, 100-101
study limitations, 107
study methods
    analytical model, 104
    data collection, 101-103
    definitions used in, 104
    treatment cost factors, 103-104
study results, 105-106
    sensitivity analyses, 106
study summary, 99-100
treatment cost statistics and,
        100,106
Diagnostic Interview Schedule for
        Children-Revised (DISC-R),
        87
Diagnostic Interview Schedule (DIS),
        101
    depression section of, 102
    depression severity, score for, 105
Diagnostic and Statistical Manual of
        Mental Disorders (DSM)
    depression symptoms and, 35
    minor and major depression
        criteria, 25,26,36
Dietrich, Allen J., 21
DIS. *See* Diagnostic Interview
        Schedule
DISC-R. *See* Diagnostic Interview
        Schedule for
        Children-Revised
DSM. *See* Diagnostic and Statistical
        Manual of Mental Disorders
DSM-III-R, 25,104
DSM-IV, 87

ECA (Epidemiologic Catchment
        Area), 1,21
Educational sectors, as gateways to
        mental health services, 83-84
Elze, Diane, 83
Emergency shelter care facility
    African-American youth and, 13
    age and, 9,12,13,15
    Asian/Pacific Islander youth and,
        13

assessments and, 8,9,17
    Caucasian youth and, 12,14,15
    child welfare system and, 6-8
    children at risk and, 8
    criminal justice systems and, 5,6,12
    emotional abuse and, 11
    emotional problems and, 87
    ethnicity and, 12,13,15
    future study directions and, 18
    gang affiliation and, 11
    gender and, 12
    Hispanic youth and, 13
    juvenile justice systems and, 5
    length of stay, 8,13
    mental health systems and, 5,6,12
    multiple system involvement, 8,87
    Native American youth and,
        12,14,15
    neglect and, 11
    older youth and, 13,15,16
    physical abuse and, 11
    physically abused youth and, 14
    placement after release, 11,13
    prior involvement of public
        services, 8,13,14,15,16,17
    sexually abused youth and, 11,14
        placement after release and, 15
    study discussion, 15-17
    study limitations, 17,18
    study methods
        intake interview, 10,11
        procedures, 9-10
        social service record reviews, 11
        subjects, 9
    study objectives, 8
    study results
        prior involvement, 11-12
        prior involvement, factors
            related to, 12-13
        prior involvement, outcomes
            relative to, 13-15
    study summary, 5-8
    substance abuse and, 11
    suicide attempts and, 11
Emotional problems. *See* Depression
Epidemiologic Catchment Area
        (ECA), 1,21

Ethnic factors
  in multiple service systems, 12-13
  See also Minority factors

Family reunification
  behavior problems and, 7,17
  preferred placement option and, 7
  shelter goal of, 8
Forty, John C., 99
Foster care system
  behavior problems and, 7,17
  mental health services and, 6,7,16

Garland, Ann F., 5
Gender factors
  children's services reactivity and,
    42,45,47,50,51,54
  in multiple service systems, 12
  See also Primary care physicians,
    physician-patient gender
    factors
General medical care sectors,
  physicians
  research needs of, 3
  See also Depression treatment;
    Primary care physicians
Glassine, Charles, 41
Guidelines for the Treatment of
    Depression in Primary Care
    (Panel, 1993), 35

Hadley-Ives, Eric, 83
Hispanic youth
  Emergency shelter facilities and, 13
  See also Minority factors

Institute of Medicine, 62,63
Interagency collaboration
  allocation of resources and, 65
  case management services and, 74
  child welfare system and, 61,65,
    67,68,70-73,76,77,78
  client referrals and, 64,67,70,77
  communication and, 64
  community-based services,
    effectiveness of 66,77
  crisis stabilization and, 74
  education linkages, 73
  financing mechanisms of, 66
  financing of, 74
  foster care and, 71,72,73,74
  funding and, 64
  group homes and, 74
  in-home intervention, 74
  information and, 64,67,71
  interagency collaboration and,
    65,66
  interagency governance structure
    and, 66,76
  joint activities and, 64
  juvenile justice systems and,
    61,65,67,68,70-73,76,77,78
  network analysis of 62,64
    rural vs. urban service network
    and, 65,68
  policies and procedures
    development and, 66
  program management and, 65
  resource exchange and, 64,65
  respite care and, 74
  service delivery problems of, 65
  structural adaptations and, 64,77
  study discussion, 76-78
  study intervention, 65-66
  study methods
    analysis procedures for, 67-69,
      79 *n. 3*
    data sources of, 66-67, 78-79
      n. 1, 79 *n. 2*
  study results
    paired linkages (specific),
      changes in, 70-73
    patterns of linkages (overall),
      changes in, 69-70
    progress reports, project
      implementation, 74-76
  study theory and, 64-65

substance abuse services and, 74,75
See also Child welfare system;
    Juvenile justice system
Interorganizational relations. *See*
    interagency collaboration

Johnsen, Matthew C., 61
Johnson, Sharon, 83
Joint Commission on the Mental
    Health of Children, 62
Juvenile justice systems
    emergency shelter care facilities
        and, 5
    emotionally disturbed children and,
        61-64
    as gateways to mental health
        services, 42,84
    interagency collaboration and,
        61,65,67,68,70-73
    network analysis and, 62
    prior involvement factors and,
        2,5,6,12

Kinship care, 7

Landsverk, John A., 5
Litrownik, Alan J., 5

Mental disorders
    burden of, 2
    detection of, 1-3
    externalizing and internalizing
        factors, 43-48,51,53,54,56,57
    See also Mental health services;
        specific disorder
Mental health services
    adolescents and, 1,6
    challenges to, 1-3,63
    child welfare system and, 2,6,84
    children and, 1,6
    communities affected by, 42

continuity of care and, 62
coordination requirements and,
    6,16
cost factors and, 2
criminal justice system and, 2,6
early problem identification and, 7
families affected by, 42
foster care and, 7
fragmentation of, 6,62
interagency collaboration and,
    61,62
juvenile justice system and, 42,84
minorities and,
    1,47,49,50,51-53,55,57
non-minorities and, 55,56,57
older adults and, 1
prior involvement and placement
    and, 2,7,44,48-49,50
rural community barriers to, 101
sectors of care and, 1-3
social service professionals and,
    83,84,85
state custody and, 41,42,56,57
Mental Health Services Program for
    Youth, of Robert Wood
    Johnson Foundation, 64,67
Minority factors
    in children's service reactivity and
        responsiveness,
        1,47,49,50,51-53,55,57
    in multiple service systems, 12-13
Morrissey, Joseph P., 61

National Association of Public Child
    Welfare Administrators, 63
National Center on Child Abuse and
    Neglect, 42
National Comorbidity Survey, 100
National Institute of Mental Health
    (NIMH), 1,3,35,85,88
National Mental Health Association,
    62
Native American youth
    Emergency shelter facilities and,
        12,14,15
    See also Minority factors

NIMH. *See* National Institute of
    Mental Health North
    Carolina Children's
    Initiative. *See* Interagency
    collaboration
Nugent, William R., 41

Office of Technology Assessment, of
    U.S. Congress, 62
Out-of-home care. *See* Foster Care
Owen, Mary, 21

Physical abuse, 6,14,42
President's Commission on Mental
    Health, 62
Primary care physicians,
    physician-patient
    gender factors and, 2,21-24
    depression and, 21-22
        detection of, 1,2,22
        diagnosis implications, 30-31
        psychosocial presentation, 22
        somatic presentation, 22
        symptoms of, 29-30
    as gateways to mental health
        services, 84
    measures of, 27-29
    medical chart notation, 33
    mental health services from, 1
    methods of analysis, 29
    procedure and data collection,
        25-27
    psychosocial stressors and, 29-30
    research focus of, 3,22
    study conclusion, 33-36
    study methods, physicians sample,
        24-25
    study results, 29-30
    study summary, 21-22
    treatment decisions, 31-33
Psychosocial problems. *See*
    Depression

QDIS. *See* Quick Diagnostic Interview
    Schedule
Quick Diagnostic Interview Schedule
    (QDIS), 104

Reiger, D.A., 1-3
Reunification policy. *See* Family
    reunification
Rivard, Jeanne C., 61
Robert Wood Johnson Foundation,
    Mental Health Services
    Program for Youth of, 64,67
    See also Interagency collaboration
Rost, Kathyyn M., 99

SACA. *See* Services Assessment for
    Children and Adolescents
Sectors of care
    community services and, 3
    general medicine and, 3
    informal care and, 3
    social services and, 3
    specialty mental health and, 3
Selective Serotonin Reuptake
    Inhibitors (SSRIs), 35
Services Assessment for Children and
    Adolescents (SACA), 87
Social service providers' roles
    age factors and, 86
    child welfare sectors and, 84-86
    client referral and, 85,86
    conduct disorders and, 84,87
    depression and, 84
        substance abuse and, 87
    educational sectors and, 83,84,85
    as gateways to mental health
        services, 83-85,90
    gender factors and, 86
    juvenile justice sectors and,
        84,85,86
    minority vs. non-minority factors
        and, 86
    primary health sectors and, 84,85,86
    psychiatrists service statistics and,
        83,85

psychologists service statistics and, 83,85
socioeconomic status and, 86
study discussion, 94-95
study methods
  analyses, 88
  design of, 85-86
  instruments of, 87
  mental health measures of, 87
  sample of, 86-87
  service use measures of, 87-88
  validation of provider
    professions, 88
study results, 89-90
  persistent problems, services for, 90-93
  profession variables in, 93-94
  quality of services factors and, 93-94
  services access, physician
    factors in, 90
  services providers and, 90-91
study summary, 83
suicidal ideation and, 87,88
Social services
  mental health services from, 1,2
  research needs in, 3
Social workers
  as mental health professionals, 3
  research focus of, 3
  service delivery systems, 3
SSRIs. *See* Selective Serotonin
  Reuptake Inhibitors

Starrett, Barbara E., 61
State Mental Health Representative for
  Children and Youth, 63
Stem, John T., 21
Stiffman, Arlene Rubin, 83
Substance abuse
  case management of, 75
  emergency shelter intake interview
    and, 11
  measures of, 87
  rural community cost offsets and, 100
  treatment and, 48,74,88
  See also Alcohol abuse
Suicide, 11,87,88

Taussig, Heather N., 5
Teacher's Report Form (TRF), 47,48
Tennessee child custody system. *See*
  Children's service systems
TRF. *See* Teacher's Report Form

Youth Services Project, 85

Zhang, Mingliang, 99